7.95

Multiple Choice Questions
in Pharmacology

Multiple Choice Questions in Pharmacology

Bryan V Robinson PhD

Senior Lecturer in Pharmacology
Guy's Hospital Medical School, London

CHURCHILL LIVINGSTONE
EDINBURGH LONDON MELBOURNE AND NEW YORK 1987

CHURCHILL LIVINGSTONE
Medical Division of Longman Group UK Limited

Distributed in the United States of America by
Churchill Livingstone Inc., 1560 Broadway, New York,
N.Y. 10036, and by associated companies, branches
and representatives throughout the world.

First published/1980
  Reprinted 1981 (Pitman Publishing Ltd)
  Reprinted 1983
  Reprinted 1984
  Reprinted 1987 (Churchill Livingstone)

ISBN 0-443-03873-2

British Library Cataloguing in Publication Data
Robinson, Bryan V
Multiple choice questions in pharmacology.
1. Drugs — Problems, exercises, etc.
I. Title
615'.1'076   RM300

Produced by Longman Group (FE) Ltd
Printed in Hong Kong

CONTENTS

INTRODUCTION

GENERAL PHARMACOLOGY

PHARMACOKINETICS

DRUG INTERACTIONS

DRUG TOXICITY

AUTONOMIC NERVOUS SYSTEM

General

Sympathetic

Parasympathetic

CONTENTS

CONTENTS

CONTENTS

INTRODUCTION

Different types of examination have different objectives and capabilities, and the greater the variety of examination the more likely it is that the overall assessment of student performance will be correct. However, irrespective of the format that is decided upon it is important that each part should be:

A Valid — measures the aspect of performance considered by the examiners to be important.

B Consistent — any student offering similar performance should receive a similar mark.

C Feasible — examinations, as much as any other part of a course, are limited by the available resources, including time available for examinations, number of students, number of staff, access to computers, etc.

Multiple choice questions (MCQs), by virtue of their objective nature and the precision with which they can be marked clearly have much to offer, especially when incorporated as part of an integrated examination scheme.

In a book designed primarily as a teaching aid for students of pharmacology (and perhaps as a source of questions for teachers), it would be inappropriate, however, to discuss at length the theory and application of student assessment. In any case, there are many books on this subject by people better qualified to discuss it than myself. Nevertheless, I would like to make a number of points which I think might be helpful to teachers contemplating the use of MCQs for both teaching and examining students of pharmacology and to the students who will face them. Much of the criticism levelled at MCQ examinations is unjustified and relates to the inadequacy, not of the system, but rather of the examiners and their use of it. As with any examination, examiners should ask a number of questions about their intentions.

What is the Purpose of the Examination?

Examinations are not just means of allocating university degrees and diplomas; a number of other functions can be fulfilled by them, and it is important to adjust the form of examination to fit the precise purpose.

To provide feedback about the course

In-course examinations provide excellent feedback to both student and teacher alike on their success so far. It will tell the student whether he or she is working hard enough, or in the right direction, and it may well motivate him or her to greater endeavour. It will likewise help the teacher to assess the success of his teaching.

MCQ examinations, because they enable a large area of the course to be covered by a relatively small examination, are particularly useful in this context. The areas where the student is lacking knowledge or where the teacher has failed to convey that knowledge are easily pinpointed and the appropriate remedy can be sought.

To provide a quality control system

The attainment of a certain minimum standard of knowledge and competence is often used as a criterion for determining whether a student should be allowed to continue to the next part of the course. This is largely the function of Part I examinations in most science degree courses, and is certainly the intention of basic medical science examinations for medical students before they continue on to their clinical studies. In the medical course it is felt that in the best interests of the patients, the clinical teachers and indeed the students themselves, that a certain minimum comprehension of the subject should have been achieved. The MCQ examination has much to recommend it in this context, but not least is the fact that a large part of the syllabus can be covered by the examination. This is especially relevant to pharmacology where it is important to have some knowledge of most types of drug.

To assess excellence

Finals examinations in honours courses or in other situations where distinctions are to be awarded require a form of assessment that will allow the students to be extended to the maximum. It is sometimes said by the ill-informed that MCQ examinations are of no value in this respect, but this is not necessarily the case. I would be the first to agree that MCQs by themselves would not fully test the student, and would give no idea of his ability to develop an argument, his practical competence, his standard of literacy or eloquence, his creativity and so on. In general, however, good students do well whatever the form of examination, and MCQs do at least give you the opportunity of discovering the breadth of their knowledge. The inclusion of MCQs in honours examinations is not something which should be dismissed out of hand.

To teach

It is said that we learn by our mistakes, but this can only happen if we realise that they are mistakes, and examinations are rarely used in this manner. This is a pity, for in theory they provide one of the most fruitful opportunities for tuition. Most students regard even in-course examinations simply as hurdles to be negotiated, and very often teachers compound this approach by simply presenting students with their marks, without discussing or analysing the answers with the students. When MCQ examinations are used the situation is even worse, because the questions are deliberately kept secret, in order to preserve the integrity of the MCQ bank. This is a great mistake for carefully chosen MCQs can provide the basis for excellent tutorials, in which the underlying importance of a particular aspect of pharmacology can be analysed in depth.

A progression from this approach is for the students to devise their own MCQs for future discussion. As anyone who has tried will vouch, it is not easy to devise MCQs that are both plausible and relevant and, since it requires an intimate working knowledge of the subject, can prove of great benefit in the teaching of pharmacology.

Which Aspects of the Course are to be Examined?

Generally speaking, the limits of any examination are automatically set by the curriculum, which in theory can represent a fairly considerable body of knowledge. In practice, however, when examiners set essay question examinations, they tend to concentrate only on the most important topics, so that just a fraction of the course is examined. Students are quick to seize upon this opportunity to reduce the amount of work required to pass an examination, and take a chance that certain topics will not appear. With MCQs this cannot happen, since it is possible to ask questions on virtually the whole syllabus in a relatively small examination. Herein lies one of the biggest pitfalls for the unwary users of MCQs, for it is easy to ask trivial and irrelevant questions, or to probe in minute detail about relatively unimportant areas of the subject. It is essential that MCQ papers like any other examination should have a suitable balance of questions, so that vital knowledge is examined thoroughly. It is a simple matter and indeed it is appropriate to include both a few easy questions, to encourage the weaker students, and a few enquiring questions, so as to extend the brighter and more well read students to the limits of their knowledge and understanding.

ADVICE TO TEACHERS

Devising MCQs

MCQ examinations provide an objective assessment of student performance with a high precision of marking accuracy. To take advantage of this, examiners must ensure that the questions are appropriate; in other words that they reflect the course in terms of both scope and degree of difficulty, that they are unambiguous and that they avoid a host of pitfalls that may reduce their usefulness (see below). Writing good questions is not easy; it takes time, practice and careful scrutiny. No matter how precise the computer analysis of the results, the assessment of student performance is only as valid as the questions which have been set.

Examiners can most easily ensure that their examination will be successful and useful by approaching question setting in a systematic fashion.

Define coverage of course

It is important to decide on:

1. Topics to be assessed, e.g. anaesthetics.
2. Areas of topic to be considered, e.g. mechanism of action, toxicity, clinical usefulness.

3

3. Depth of knowledge expected, e.g. concentrations required to induce anaesthesia, solubility in blood, partial pressures.

4. Whether examination is to test factual information or terminology, or the students' problem-solving abilities (or all of these).

Determine form of questions

Medical MCQs are invariably of the multiple true/false (independent) format where any number of the alternatives may be correct. This type of question is used primarily because of the difficulty of finding four plausible distractors when the one from five system is used. Each question consists of a stem and a number of statements (usually five) relating to this.

The stem may be:

1. a single word, e.g. **ether.**
2. a phrase, e.g. **'Complications associated with the use of ether include . . .'** or, **'Which of the following statements is/are correct . . .'**
3. a problem, e.g. **'When injected into a young adult a drug causes a fall in blood pressure, a dilated pupil and a dry mouth.'** or **'The drug . . .'**
4. Photographs, ecgs, X-rays and biochemical data are often included in the stem of questions in many medical disciplines, but these are less easily used in pharmacology.

The statements relating to the stem may be either a single word (e.g. atropine, tachycardia, increase) or a phrase (e.g. is contraindicated in anxiety states).

Write individual questions

MCQs must be unequivocal in their wording and to be sure of this, it is advisable to follow a few simple rules.

1. Be specific. If there is any possibility that species, age, sex, route of administration etc. will influence the effect of a drug then be quite categorical about this in the question.

Example: **Injection of adrenaline characteristically produces**
              A a fall in blood pressure.

This is a bad question, because it does not define the species, the route of injection or whether systolic or diastolic blood pressure is being considered. Typically, subcutaneous injection of adrenaline in man produces a fall in diastolic pressure, whilst intravenous injection into the cat causes a rise.

Wherever possible be quantitative rather than qualitative, but if a figure cannot be placed on the incidence of a feature then use words such as *characteristic* or *typical* for features that occur so frequently as to be expected, and *recognised* or *accepted* for features that, although not characteristic, may sometimes occur.

2. Avoid ambiguity

(a) Double negatives (one in the stem and one in the statement) should never be used and single negatives avoided except where their removal might defeat the intention of the question.

(b) Words like 'always, never,' should not be used, because in medicine there are usually exceptions and the bright student will enter FALSE to such a statement.

(c) Check that the question is grammatically correct, and that it does not give inadvertent clues as to the number of correct alternatives or to which alternative is correct.

3. Select alternatives with care. Apart from selecting alternatives that are feasible and that are either categorically right or wrong, it is important in the independent true/false type of question to ensure that selection of a particular alternative does not modify a student's approach to other alternatives.

Example: **Acetylcholine**
                A increases heart rate
                B decreases heart rate

These are mutually exclusive alternatives, so that a student who gets it right will get a bonus mark, whereas one who gets it wrong is doubly penalised. Phrases such as 'all of these' or 'none of these' similarly have no place; this type of answer is suitable only for the one from five type of question.

Look at the overall format of examinations

Having spent time and effort in devising good individual questions, it is important to ensure that the completed examination has the correct balance and to this end the examiner should again ask himself a few pertinent questions.

1. Are the questions testing what is being taught?
2. Is the 'mix' of questions from different areas correct?
3. Do the questions overlap?
4. Are the questions of the appropriate degree of difficulty with both easy and difficult questions to encourage the weak and to stretch the capable? It should be remembered in this context that only difficult questions have the ability to discriminate between good and bad students (*see* page 7).

Scrutinise the final product

Once the appropriate questions have been compiled into an examination, instructions to students must be added (including the time allocated for the examination) and the final copy diligently proof-read to remove spelling and transcription errors. Finally, the examination should be read by a colleague who has not been involved in compiling the examination.

Analysis of results

A detailed description of the computer analysis of examination results would not be appropriate, but there are a few essential features of the print-out which deserve a brief mention in order that the examination may be used in the most fruitful fashion. A reader requiring further information should consult one of the books given in the further reading list.

Assessment of students

Student performance can be judged in two ways; in terms of rank and in terms of a specific mark. Rank is a self-explanatory term, but provides an amazingly accurate, though qualitative, estimate of student performance. There is generally very good agreement in the ranking of both bright and poor students when assessed by essay and by MCQ examinations; although the correlation may be less obvious with the middle range students.

Probably the most acceptable quantitative assessment of student performance is given by the corrected percentage score. This is calculated from the formula:

$$\text{Corrected percentage score} = \frac{\text{Raw Score} \times 100}{\text{maximum possible score}}$$

$$\text{Where Raw Score} = \left(\begin{array}{c} \text{Number of} \\ \text{correct} \\ \text{'yes'} \\ \text{responses} \end{array} + \begin{array}{c} \text{Number of} \\ \text{correct} \\ \text{'no'} \\ \text{responses} \end{array} \right) - \left(\begin{array}{c} \text{Number of} \\ \text{incorrect} \\ \text{'yes'} \\ \text{responses} \end{array} + \begin{array}{c} \text{Number of} \\ \text{incorrect} \\ \text{'no'} \\ \text{responses} \end{array} \right)$$

This formula takes account of guessing and for a student to achieve a mark at all he must get more than 50 per cent of the responses correct.

Marks obtained in this way have a wider spread (typically between 20 to 80 per cent) than those obtained by the 'close-marking' system commonly adopted for essay examinations. Furthermore, the pass mark is not necessarily 50 per cent and must be set by the examiner after careful scrutiny of the questions. The precise positioning of the pass mark will depend on the degree of difficulty of the questions and the level of expected attainment of the students. The examiner may find it helpful in this respect to plot a histogram of student marks in order to identify the clearly good and bad students.

If the examiner wishes to combine marks from MCQ examinations and other examinations, and the two sets of marks are to carry the same weight, it is essential that the marks should be spread over a similar range. There are various manoeuvres for doing this, but I favour the system which first sets the pass mark using the corrected percentage scores. This may be put at, say 56 per cent, but in the calculation that follows will be transposed to the conventional 50 per cent. The bright students are then identified and the top marks normally awarded in essay questions designated to correspond to the top marks of the MCQ examination (e.g. an MCQ mark of 75 per cent might become 60 per cent on the close marking scheme). A linear regression plot is then calculated, using these two sets of marks, either with the aid of a desk calculator, or by plotting the results graphically. In any event, the remaining marks may be similarly transposed.

If the examiner has any doubt concerning the unexpected failure of a particular student, then until he gains experience with the system he should hand-mark a few papers, noting the responses to individual questions to check that the pass mark is indeed failing and passing at the correct point. Furthermore, even with considerable experience of the system, it is wise to check the papers of students where there are major discrepancies between essay and MCQ marks. A large difference may be traceable to a particular underlying cause (e.g. omission of an essay question).

Assessment of questions

There are two important indices that can be derived from an analysis of the responses made by students in a particular examination.

1. Facility index (F). This is simply the percentage or fraction of students who make the correct response for a particular item in a given question. Thus, if four-fifths of the students answer an item correctly, then F = 80 per cent (or 0.80). It must be remembered, of course, that the ease with which students answer a question is dependent not just on the relative simplicity of the question, but also on their state of knowledge regarding the subject being examined. A question relating to an area of pharmacology not covered by the syllabus may appear difficult to the students even though the concepts involved are relatively facile.

A good examination will contain some easy and some difficult questions, but the easier the question the less useful it becomes as a means of discriminating between students (see below).

2. Discrimination index. This is a measure of how useful a particular item is in distinguishing the clever students from the not so clever. It is calculated by looking at the performance in answering a particular item of the top group of students (as assessed by their position in the whole examination), and comparing it with the performance of the bottom group of students. Various procedures may be adopted, comparing different fractions of the student population taking the examination, e.g. the top half with the bottom half or the top 27 per cent with the bottom 27 per cent. The index can be calculated from simple ratios of correct answers in each group, or by using more complex statistical evaluations of the expected and actual incidence of correct answers in each group (e.g. involving a Chi-squared test).

Whichever technique is used, a positive index will result from questions that can discriminate between good and bad students, the higher the index the better the discrimination. The precise value will depend on the method of calculation, but is generally within the range 0.05 to 0.5.

For an examination to be of real value an average discrimination within the middle of this range would be advisable. This in turn means that only a few very easy questions should be included because the discrimination indices of easy questions (i.e. ones with a facility index of 0.95 or over) are low and generally less reliable. This is because in a total entry of say 100 candidates, only 2 or 3 students in each group are being compared.

7

Any question in which a negative discrimination is produced should be scrutinised carefully. It may be due to an incorrect entry on the master answer sheet which has been used to programme the marking by computer. However, in this case, the question would appear to be very difficult (i.e. have a low facility index). It is more likely that the question has been poorly constructed or is simply ambiguous. For example, in the item, 'α-blockers are used in the treatment of essential hypertension' average and below average students will probably realise that in general, this is not the case and enter FALSE, whilst brighter students may realise that the antihypertensive drug prazosin may be effective because of its ability to block specifically postsynaptic α-receptors, and enter TRUE. If the computer has been programmed to accept FALSE as the correct answer, then it is likely that a negative discrimination index will result. Such questions must either by rewritten in an unequivocal fashion (e.g. the α-blocker phentolamine is used in the treatment of essential hypertension) or abandoned altogether.

ADVICE TO STUDENTS

Preparation

The preparation required for MCQ examinations is essentially similar to that required for any other form of examination, namely to be aware of the syllabus, to know the priorities within it, and to have sufficient knowledge to satisfy the examiners.

MCQ examinations primarily test the vocabulary of the subject and specific factual knowledge. To a lesser extent, they test interpretation of facts and the ability to solve problems. They do not test at all the ability to expound an argument and they are not influenced by literary style or grammatical ineptitude (except of the examiner). Students who are conscious of the importance of such aspects of examination technique can often tip the balance in their favour when answering essay questions, but will have no such control when answering MCQs. On the other hand, less eloquent students or ones with poor handwriting who may fare less favourably at the hand of the examiner will be treated equally impartially by MCQs (whether marked by hand or by computer).

Although no special revision is required for MCQ examinations, as with all styles of examination, some practice beforehand can only be an advantage. After all, the examination is intended to test your knowledge of pharmacology, not your familiarity (or lack of it) with the MCQ system. Unfortunately for students, most MCQs are held in University or College question banks and are not freely available for revision purposes. Such secrecy is imposed partly by University or College rules and partly by the problems of setting a sufficient number of pertinent, plausible and generally well designed questions.

However, in my opinion, MCQs when accompanied by answers and explanations provide an excellent system for self-tuition and for revision, and it is hoped that this book will not only familiarise the student with MCQs in pharmacology, but also help to fill gaps in his or her knowledge.

Answering MCQs

It is likely that in a qualifying examination the paper will be marked by computer, and since this is not endowed with the gift of insight into students' intentions that many examiners have, it is important that candidates follow the instructions to the letter.

Most of the business of entering information on the MCQ answer sheets is commonsense, but it is important to get it right. To assist in this process the various steps are set out below with some advice on the decisions you are making.

1. At the risk of repeating myself, read carefully the instructions to candidates and follow them.

2. Enter your name, test number, college number, candidate number etc. both by marks in the matrix and in writing (to enable your paper to be identified if you enter the numbers incorrectly in the matrix).

3. Mark your responses in the appropriate boxes on the answer sheet. This invariably requires the use of an HB pencil in order that the marks can be scored by the computer.

(A) for a 'yes' response (TRUE)
(A) for a 'no' response (FALSE)

Make a *neat but positive* vertical line in the box of your choice. If you change your mind, erase the mistake and try again. The computer is arranged to record the more positive of two marks. DO NOT play Russian roulette by making barely visible lines or by entering marks of similar intensity into both boxes, leaving the computer to decide your intention. Also make sure that you are marking the correct answer box (i.e. yes or no) and that the number corresponds to the question number.

4. Remember the marking system

Correct answers	+ 1 mark
Incorrect answers	− 1 mark
No attempt	0 mark

This system is used to give students (especially of medicine) the opportunity to admit ignorance, on the basis that it is better to recognise this fact than to do something incorrectly (e.g. administer potentially dangerous drugs inappropriately). In the practical terms of answering MCQs, however, if you make a guess at each item (based on *no* knowledge of pharmacology) then you have a 50 : 50 chance of getting an item right (or wrong). If you were to approach the whole examination like that, you would statistically expect to achieve a zero score, which is no better than one would expect if a man in the street were invited to sit the examination. On the other hand, not answering a particular item (so avoiding a possible penalty mark) would also give you a zero score, and clearly if you do not attempt a large number of questions (say 30 per cent of the total) you will automatically reduce the total score which you can possibly achieve, and therefore your chances of passing the examination. In terms, therefore, of achieving the maximum possible score in an examination, judicious guessing based on some knowledge of the subject may be advisable. The option of omission is really intended as a way of escaping a penalty mark in a few answers where you are completely stumped.

5. Read the questions carefully. Many medical terms, drug names, nomenclatures, etc. sound and/or look very similar.

e.g. increase/decrease, β_1/β_2, systolic/diastolic, tachycardia/bradycardia, effective/ineffective

It is foolish to throw away marks because of misreading.

FURTHER READING

ANDERSON, J. (1976) *The multiple choice question in medicine.* London: Pitman Medical.

HARDEN, R. McG. (1979) Constructing multiple choice questions of the multiple true/false type. *Medical Education,* **13,** 305–312. (Available as Medical Education Booklet No. 10 from Association for the Study of Medical Education. 150b Perth Road, Dundee, DD1 4EA).

An Introduction and Guide to the Use of Multiple Choice Questions in University Examinations. University of London, 1976.

ACKNOWLEDGEMENTS

To devise 250 original and acceptable multiple choice questions (MCQs) is a formidable task for one person, and it will come as no surprise to the reader to learn that many of the MCQs in this book come from a departmental bank of questions which has developed over a number of years. They have been written by various members of staff, and I am grateful to Frank House, Paul Morrison, Howard Rogers, Frank Sullivan and Roy Spector for permission to use them in the book. I trust they will forgive the way in which some of them have been combined and mutilated.

I would also like to thank my friend and colleague Frank Sullivan for his assistance and encouragement in the project, my wife Christina for the many hours of typing to produce the manuscript, various colleagues at Guy's and elsewhere who have been kind enough to read and comment on sections of the book, and the staff of Pitman Medical for their help in producing the book so quickly and efficiently.

1 Which of the following drug combinations demonstrate 'physiological antagonism'

    A isoprenaline and histamine on the bronchioles
    B isoprenaline and propranolol on the bronchioles
    C isoprenaline and SRS-A on the bronchioles
    D acetylcholine and adrenaline on the heart
    E phenylephrine and physostigmine on the pupil

Note: Physiological antagonism is said to occur when one drug overcomes the effect of another; not by displacing it from the receptor sites (which is competitive antagonism), but by stimulating totally different receptors to produce the opposite effect.

A TRUE In the bronchioles isoprenaline stimulates β_2-receptors to induce dilatation whilst histamine stimulates H_1-receptors to cause constriction.

B FALSE Propranolol is a competitive antagonist of the actions of isoprenaline (both β_1 and β_2) throughout the body.

C TRUE Slow reacting substance of anaphylaxis (SRS-A) is a potent constrictor of bronchioles that is released from mast cells in the lungs of asthmatic subjects. Isoprenaline by stimulating β_2-receptors induces dilatation and is useful in symptomatic treatment of this condition.

D TRUE Acetylcholine by stimulating muscarinic receptors especially in the sinoatrial node reduces heart rate and force of contraction. Adrenaline by stimulating β-receptors increases both the rate and force of contraction.

E TRUE Phenylephrine is an α-stimulant which dilates the pupil by causing contractions of the smooth muscle of the dilator pupillae. Physostigmine is a cholinesterase inhibitor which potentiates the pupillary constrictor action of the normally released acetylcholine. It does this by preventing the breakdown of that acetylcholine which then acts on muscarinic receptors to effect contraction of the smooth muscle of the constrictor pupillae.

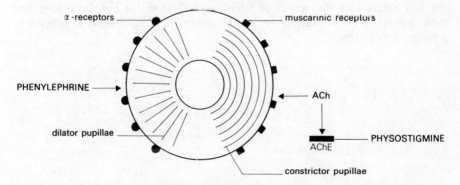

2 Which of the following pairs of drugs compete for the same receptors

    A strychnine and glycine
    B cimetidine and histamine
    C benzhexol and acetylcholine
    D haloperidol and dopamine
    E morphine and noradrenaline

A TRUE Glycine is a postsynaptic inhibitory transmitter at spinal motoneurones. Its action is selectively blocked by strychnine, the results of which are an increase in the motor effects of spinal reflexes and a reduced latent period. Large doses of strychnine send all the voluntary muscles in the body into spasms to produce violent, painful convulsions.

B TRUE Cimetidine is an H_2-receptor blocker and therefore competes with histamine in the stomach to prevent gastric acid release, in the myocardium to prevent the chronotropic action of histamine and on the rat uterus to inhibit histamine-induced contractions.

C TRUE Benzhexol is a blocker of the muscarinic actions of acetylcholine. It is used in the treatment of Parkinson's disease, because it reduces the cholinergic dominance that follows depletion of dopamine in the nigrostriatal pathway. It controls the rigidity of the disease, but as might be expected its use is accompanied by anticholinergic problems, e.g. dry mouth, blurred vision, etc.

D TRUE Haloperidol is a butyrophenone with powerful antipsychotic activity. It is a receptor antagonist of dopamine which is thought to be the mechanism of its antipsychotic action, but by preventing dopamine action in the corpus striatum it also causes Parkinsonian side effects.

E FALSE The actions of morphine on the cns may be explained largely in terms of its ability to bind to the same receptors to which enkephalins (naturally occurring pentapeptides) bind. These receptors have been described as opiate receptors. There is also evidence that morphine interferes with cholinergic transmission in the cns and antagonises the action of 5-hydroxytryptamine at peripheral sites, but there appears to be no evidence for competition with noradrenaline at either α or β-adrenoceptor sites.

3 Which of the following statements is/are correct

    A drug receptor interactions generally involve covalent binding
    B nicotine is a partial agonist
    C the sympathetic supply to the sweat glands is cholinergic
    D antagonists dissociate slowly from receptors
    E β-receptor stimulation typically causes inhibition of adenyl cyclase

A FALSE Drugs are in general bound to receptors by a variety of weak electrical bonds including electrostatic forces, London dispersion forces (Van de Waal's forces), and hydrogen binding, all of which allow relatively rapid movement of the molecule on and off the receptor. Covalent binding of drugs to receptors is uncommon and results in a more stable and much longer lasting effect. Examples of covalent binding include alkylation of DNA by antimitotic agents and phosphorylation of cholinesterase by organophosphorus compounds.

B TRUE Partial agonists are substances which on contact with a receptor initially stimulate it (agonist action) but then by remaining attached to the receptor effectively prevent the action of other drugs (antagonist action). Nicotine has this effect at autonomic ganglia.

C TRUE Although sympathetic nerves are characteristically noradrenergic, the transmitter at the sympathetic nerves supplying the sweat glands is acetylcholine.

D TRUE According to the rate theory of drug action, agonist molecules dissociate from receptors rapidly providing a large number of free receptors for subsequent interactions. Antagonists on the other hand dissociate from the receptor slowly, thereby reducing the number of free receptors and hence the possible number of reactions with agonist molecules.

E FALSE It has been shown that many of the actions of β-adrenoceptor stimulants are accompanied by a rise in intracellular cyclic AMP (cAMP) levels, brought about by *increased* activity of adenyl cyclase in the cell membrane. It is widely believed that β-stimulants bring about an allosteric change in the enzyme such that increased catabolic activity occurs.

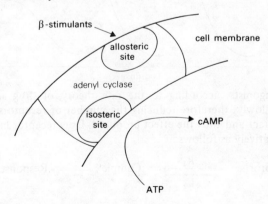

4 Competitive antagonists

    A dissociate from receptors faster than their respective agonists
    B alter the shape of the log dose response curve of an agonist
    C according to the rate theory have low dissociation rate constants
    D are selective drugs that will block only one receptor type e.g. H_1-receptors
    E initiate the opposite cellular response to receptor occupancy to that obtained by the agonist

---

A FALSE According to the rate theory of drug action a drug molecule only produces an effect at the moment of interaction with a receptor. Thus substances which associate and dissociate with receptors very rapidly are agonists because this leaves a large number of receptors available for further interactions. Substances which dissociate from the receptors slowly, on the other hand, reduce the possible number of drug receptor interactions in a given time and are therefore termed antagonists.

B FALSE Competitive antagonists as their name suggests compete with the corresponding agonist molecules for a place on the receptor. The success of a particular molecular species in producing its effect will be dependent on its relative affinity for the receptor and the total number of molecules of that type in the receptor area (i.e. molar concentration). Measurement of the dose-response relationship of a particular agonist in the presence of a competitive antagonist will not therefore prevent a normal maximum response from being achieved (i.e. the antagonism can be overcome). The dose-response curve is simply shifted to the right. With insurmountable (non-competitive) antagonism the size of maximal effect would be reduced.

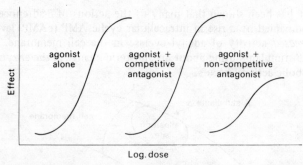

C TRUE Antagonists, according to the rate theory of drug action, dissociate from receptors slowly, therefore reducing the number of receptors with which the agonist can interact and thus the effect produced. Drug receptor interaction can be expressed qualitatively as follows:

$$\text{Drug} + \text{Receptor} \xrightleftharpoons[k_2]{k_1} \text{Complex} \longrightarrow \text{Response}$$

Rate of association $= k_1 (1-y) A$
Rate of dissociation $= k_2 y$

At equilibrium

$$k_1 (1-y)A = k_2 y$$

A = drug concentration
y = proportion of receptors occupied
k_1 = association rate constant
k_2 = dissociation rate constant

Thus if k_2 is large the rate of dissociation is high then the drug is an agonist, but if k_2 is small the drug comes off slowly (reducing the available receptors) and is an antagonist.

D FALSE The degree of specificity demonstrated by antagonists tends to be greater than that shown by agonists and whilst histamine stimulates both H_1 and H_2-receptors, mepyramine antagonises only H_1 effects. On the other hand, mepyramine also has weak anticholinergic activity and the ability to antagonise (be it all less powerfully) another receptor type is a feature of many antagonists.

E FALSE Competitive antagonists bind to the same receptors as the corresponding agonist. Characteristically, they do not invoke a cellular response, although some antagonists may have weak agonistic activity. They are then termed partial agonists. A substance that produces the opposite cellular response will do so by stimulating different receptors and is termed a physiological antagonist.

5 Two different choline esters when added independently to an isolated smooth muscle preparation (guinea pig ileum) produced quantitatively similar contractions of the muscle. It is implicit that both drugs

    A occupy the same number of receptors
    B are present in similar molar concentration
    C have similar affinity constants
    D will be antagonised by atropine
    E will be antagonised by iodoacetate

A FALSE The extent of the effect produced by any given drug is the result not only of the number of receptors with which it interacts, but also with the outcome of that interaction. Thus one drug with high efficacy may produce maximal effect when occupying only a few receptors, whilst another with lower efficacy by occupying a greater number of receptors will achieve the same response.

B FALSE Implicit in the idea that the number and nature of the drug-receptor interactions is responsible for the extent of effect (see A) is the fact that similar responses can be achieved with different molar concentrations of the drug in the vicinity of the receptors.

C FALSE The affinity (or equilibrium constant) of a drug is the ratio of the association rate constant (k_1) divided by the dissociation rate constant (k_2).

Rate of association $= k_1 (1-y)A$
Rate of dissociation $= k_2 y$

At equilibrium

$$\text{Affinity constant } (K_A) = \frac{k_1}{k_2} = \frac{y}{(1-y)A}$$

From this formula it can be seen that if two drugs produce similar actions then only if their molar concentration and degree of receptor occupancy are the same would their affinity constants be similar, and this may not be the case (see A and B).

D FALSE This may not be the case because smooth muscle of the ileum is supplied with both nicotinic and muscarinic receptors and a drug with exclusively nicotinic actions will not be antagonised by atropine.

E TRUE Receptors provide the interface between a drug and the activation processes of a cell (e.g. muscle contraction) and a number of different receptor types can gain access to the same system (e.g. acetylcholine, histamine, nicotine, etc.). In the case of an homologous series of compounds they will all interact with the same receptor type. However iodoacetate is an inhibitor of energy supply within the cell and will antagonise muscle contraction induced by both drugs.

6 In the laboratory testing of new drugs

A the LD_{50} (rats) of a drug is the dose that will kill 50 per cent of the rats injected

B information on carcinogenicity of compounds is obtained from acute toxicity tests

C teratogenicity tests examine the potential of a drug to produce congenital abnormalities if given during pregnancy

D the carcinogenic potential of a drug is obvious when administered for about one third of the lifespan of an animal

E the therapeutic index is an indication of the potency of a drug

---

A TRUE The LD_{50} or median lethal dose of a drug is the amount (in mg/kg) which kills half of a group of animals. It can be calculated from a plot of lethality against the logarithm of dose over a range of doses.

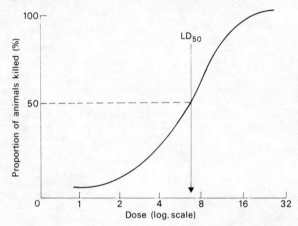

B FALSE Acute toxicity tests involve giving each animal a single injection of the drug but using several groups of animals so that the LD_{50} can be calculated (see A). Acute toxicity tests will give the first indication of probable toxicity problems, but because they last only about seven days will give no indication of carcinogenicity (see D).

C TRUE Teratology is the science which has developed since the thalidomide disaster to study the possible action of drugs on the developing fetus if given during pregnancy. The studies are commonly performed in the rat or mouse, and involve giving the drug to the animal from at least the first day of pregnancy until just before term.

D FALSE The risk that a neoplasm will develop following exposure to a drug is dependent amongst other factors on the length of time over which the drug is administered, and the latent period of the developing cancer. Thus if a drug is to be administered over a large proportion of the individual's lifespan and mainly during the early part of his life, the possibility that a carcinogenic action will be produced increases. It is essential therefore when studying the possible carcinogenic action of a drug to expose the animals to the drug from weaning and to continue the study throughout the major part of their lives.

E FALSE The therapeutic index is the ratio of the dose of a drug which is just toxic (maximum tolerated dose) and that which is just effective (minimum effective dose). The larger the ratio then the greater will be the margin of safety. An estimate of the therapeutic index can be obtained experimentally from the ratio of LD_{50} : ED_{50}, i.e. median lethal dose (see A) : median effective dose.

7 New drugs in the United Kingdom

A may be sold by pharmacies only after a product licence has been issued by the Medicines Commission

B may be used in patients by hospital doctors before a licence is issued

C must be approved by the EEC

D must be shown to be non-carcinogenic before a product licence will be issued irrespective of the manner of administration or the disease condition to be treated

E can only be licensed if their mechanism of action has been clearly elucidated

---

A TRUE Under the Medicines Act (1968) all medicines (except those appearing on a general sales list) must be sold from registered pharmacies and new drugs can only be sold in this way after the issue of a product licence by the Medicines Commission.

B FALSE The Medicines Act (1968) controls by the issuing of licences the marketing, importation and production of medicines for human (and veterinary) use. The purpose of the Act is primarily to protect the public against avoidable hazards which might arise from the introduction of a new therapeutic agent. Before a clinical trial can be carried out whether in general practice, a general hospital or a teaching hospital, the Committee on Safety of Medicines (CSM) must be satisfied, on the basis of submitted evidence, that the drug is effective and does not in animals demonstrate undue toxicity.

C FALSE At present it is only necessary to satisfy the UK licensing authorities but no doubt as greater legislative unity takes place within the Common Market, EEC approval will become necessary.

D FALSE Tests for carcinogenicity constitute an essential part of any submission to the CSM, and whilst an oral contraceptive which has been shown to produce an increased incidence of cancer in experimental animals would not be approved, an anticancer drug with a similar action would almost certainly be licensed. The decision is one based on the risks and benefits of any particular drug within the context of its intended use.

E FALSE If this were the case, it is probable that no new drugs would be introduced. Although information is often available on the likely mechanism of action of a drug before it is marketed, absence of this information would certainly not prevent the granting of a product licence. After decades on the market the precise mechanism of action of many drugs is still far from clear, especially those acting on the central nervous system.

8 Before conducting a clinical trial on a new drug in the United Kingdom

A it is mandatory to obtain permission from the Medicines Commission
B information on toxicity in animals must be available
C the effect of the drug on pregnant animals should normally have been tested
D evidence concerning the potential cost of the drug must be submitted
E evidence concerning the need for a new drug must be submitted, i.e. currently available drugs and their efficacy

---

Note: Before the thalidomide tragedy drug companies could produce and market new drugs without seeking approval from other independent or state authorities. In 1968, the Medicines Act established a Licensing Authority for the marketing, importation and manufacture of medicines for human and veterinary use; and it is now mandatory to seek the approval of the Committee on the Safety of Medicines (CSM) at various stages during the introduction of new drugs.

A TRUE A drug company wishing to carry out clinical trials on a new drug must first submit information on the pharmacology, toxicity, teratogenicity, metabolism, etc. to the CSM. This information is reviewed by members of the subcommittees on toxicity, clinical trials and therapeutic efficacy and adverse reactions. The function of the CSM is two-fold, namely to assess the adequacy of the data submitted and the fitness of the drug for administration to man. A trials certificate will be issued if the submission meets with approval; if not, further work may be required.

B TRUE As part of the submission for permission to carry out a clinical trial (see A) information on toxicity in animals is required. The precise design of the tests performed will be dependent on such factors as the nature of the drug, its proposed use and the duration and route of administration. Generally at least two species, including a non-rodent, would be studied.

C TRUE As part of the general study of drug toxicity an investigation of the action of the drug on pregnant animals is required. This is to assess possible interference with pregnancy and particularly the production of abnormalities of fetal development.

D FALSE The CSM is not concerned with the cost of a new drug. This is determined by such things as development costs, potential sales, cost of alternative preparations etc., and will be set by the drug company.

E FALSE The question of whether there is a need for a new drug in a particular treatment area again does not fall within the purview of the CSM. The committee is concerned only with efficacy and safety. It is necessary to prove only that the drug is more effective than no treatment, not that it is more effective than an existing treatment (provided of course it is not more toxic). In any case in terms of commercial viability, submissions made to the CSM are generally for drugs in areas of therapy where effective non-toxic drugs do not already exist.

9 In the investigations relating to the introduction of a new drug, which of the following is/are true

    A only drugs with a therapeutic ratio in excess of 5 will be granted a product licence

    B double blind trials refer to the procedure in which a drug and a placebo are administered to each of two patients for a given period and then the drugs are switched by the doctor without the knowledge of the patient

    C once a drug has been given a product licence it falls outside the jurisdiction of the CSM

    D the therapeutic index is a register of all drugs which have been passed by the Committee on Safety of Medicines (CSM)

    E sequential analysis is a method of statistical evaluation of drug efficacy that enables the trial to be stopped at the earliest opportunity

---

A FALSE Therapeutic ratio is the same as therapeutic index and refers to the ratio between the dose of the drug which is just toxic (maximum tolerated dose) and that which is just effective (minimum effective dose). The larger the ratio the greater is the margin of safety. Whilst it is desirable to have a drug with a high ratio it is not essential. A value in excess of 5 would certainly be required for example for a hypnotic, which, because of its central action and the manner of administration may lead to accidental overdosage. Nevertheless, many drugs given under close supervision have smaller ratios and some anticancer drugs have a therapeutic index approaching unity. The granting of a product licence takes into account the proposed manner of administration.

B FALSE A double blind trial refers to those clinical investigations of new drugs in which the identity of the active drug or drugs and of the placebo is withheld from both the patients and the physician (and any observer if not the physician). This is to avoid psychological influences and observer bias which such information may impart. Changing over the therapy between the groups of patients in a trial (with or without their knowledge) is known as a cross-over design and helps to reduce the variability of the trial.

C FALSE The Adverse Reactions Subcommittee of the CSM collate information from a number of sources (e.g. doctors, dentists, coroners), and keep a central register of adverse reactions. Should a new drug in general use show undue toxicity then warnings or limitations about its use may be issued. If potentially fatal disorders (e.g. blood dyscrasias) or frankly harmful reactions (e.g. blindness) occur, the product licence may be withdrawn.

D FALSE See A.

E TRUE In conventional trials in which patients are allocated to particular treatment groups of specific size, it is usually necessary to complete the treatment course before the data can be analysed, and before the efficacy of one drug compared with another can be evaluated. With sequential trials patients are entered into the trial as they become available, and either two treatments are compared in one patient or between two patients, to establish which is better. If an excess preference for one treatment develops it becomes apparent as the trial proceeds and as soon as a certain predetermined level of statistical significance is exceeded the trial can be stopped.

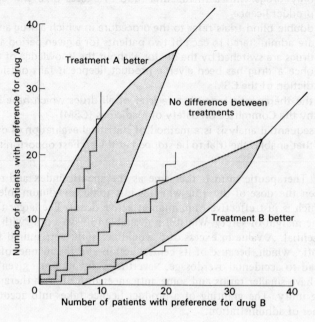

GENERAL PHARMACOLOGY

10 Which of the following statements is/are correct

A ketamine is used in the treatment of migraine
B acute systemic anaphylaxis should be treated immediately by intravenous injection of adrenaline (1 ml of 1 : 1000)
C sulphonylureas are oral anticoagulants
D procainamide is metabolised more slowly than procaine
E ethosuximide is a bacteriostatic antimicrobial drug

A FALSE Ketamine is an intravenous anaesthetic that is used to produce a state of dissociative anaesthesia in which the patient appears to be awake yet is unaware of his surroundings.

B FALSE The drug and dose are correct, but it should be administered subcutaneously. The adrenaline helps to reverse the pulmonary and cardiovascular effects of the histamine liberated into the circulation.

C FALSE Sulphonylureas (e.g. tolbutamide) are orally active antidiabetic drugs. They work by increasing the release of insulin from the pancreas.

D TRUE The local anaesthetic procaine has a stabilising (quinidine-like) action on cardiac muscle. However, it is rapidly broken down in the circulation by plasma pseudocholinesterase to para-amino-benzoic acid (PABA) and diethyl-amino-ethanol. The amide of procaine is resistant to cholinesterase and when given intravenously has a useful antidysrhythmic action.

E FALSE Ethosuximide is a succinimide used in the treatment of 'petit mal' epilepsy.

General Pharmacology: related questions 37, 44, 53, 54, 159, 160, 161, 192

11 Characteristically following oral administration to man, drugs

    A are absorbed more readily when in the unionised rather than in the ionised form

    B with high affinity for circulating protein have a high rate of urinary excretion

    C are absorbed primarily in the intestine

    D cross membranes mainly by simple diffusion

    E with high lipid solubility readily penetrate into the cns

---

A TRUE The transfer of electrolytes through lipid membranes is by simple diffusion (see D) of the unionised species. The degree of ionisation of a particular substance is dependent on its pK and the pH of the environment around the membrane: the rate of transport through the membrane will then depend on such factors as the lipid solubility, molecular weight and molecular configuration of the unionised molecule. These factors determine the diffusion constant (K) of a drug (see D).

B FALSE Glomerular filtration in the kidney allows quite large molecules to pass into the tubular lumen (e.g. haemoglobin, molecular weight 68,000), but unless there is damage to the kidney, plasma proteins do not normally find their way into the urine. Substances bound to plasma proteins similarly remain in the bloodstream and, although as free drug is removed from the plasma the equilibrium is upset, drugs with high affinity for plasma protein are slowly excreted in the urine.

C TRUE The primary site of absorption of most drugs following oral administration is the small intestine. Only alcohol and weak acids like salicylates are absorbed to any extent in the stomach. The latter, because of their pK, are in the unionised condition at gastric pH which makes them available for absorption.

D TRUE Most drugs cross membranes by simple diffusion, moving down a concentration gradient until the drug becomes evenly distributed on both sides of the membrane, or until other factors (e.g. removal by blood, excretion, metabolism) disturb the equilibrium.

The rate of diffusion can be expressed by the following formula:

$$\text{Rate} = K \; \frac{A\,(C_1 - C_2)}{d}$$

$C_1 - C_2$ = concentration gradient
d = thickness of membrane
A = surface area available
K = diffusion constant (see A)

E TRUE One of the most important factors in determining the rate of movement of drugs into tissues is the lipid solubility of that agent. In areas like the brain with high lipid content this becomes even more relevant, and explains the very rapid uptake into the brain of the highly lipid soluble agent thiopentone.

12 Which of the following statements concerning drug absorption is/are correct

    A aspirin is absorbed in the stomach
    B enteric-coated tablets are used to avoid destruction of a drug by gastric juices
    C isoprenaline is destroyed in the gastrointestinal tract following oral administration
    D the presence of milk in the gastrointestinal tract *decreases* the absorption of tetracyclines
    E the presence of milk in the gastrointestinal tract *increases* the absorption of griseofulvin

---

A **TRUE** Absorption of drugs in the stomach depends primarily on the proportion of unionised molecules present, and their lipid solubility. The extent of ionisation is dependent in turn on the pK of the drug (for aspirin about 4) and the pH of the environment.

$$\text{Since } pK = pH + \text{Log} \frac{[HA]}{[A^-]}$$

In the stomach at pH 2

$$4 = 2 + \text{Log} \frac{[HA]}{[A^-]}$$

$$\text{Log} \frac{[HA]}{[A^-]} = 2 \qquad\qquad \text{i.e. } \frac{100}{1} = 1 \text{ per cent}$$

Thus aspirin at gastric pH is only 1 per cent ionised and can therefore be absorbed, although the extent of absorption is dependent on other factors like rate of gastric emptying, solubility of the aspirin, presence of food, etc.

B **TRUE** Enteric-coated tablets are covered in a layer of shellac or gelatin to prevent the immediate dissolution of the tablet on entering the stomach. In theory, the layer is slowly dissolved by the gastric acid to liberate the contents when it passes into the duodenum. This protects both the tablet from destruction by gastric juices and the stomach lining from possible harmful effects of the drug. In practice such drugs are unreliable. Pitting of the outer covering may release the drug before it leaves the stomach, or the coating may remain round the drug so that little or none is absorbed.

C **TRUE** Isoprenaline given orally is readily broken down by catechol-O-methyl transferase (COMT) in both the gastrointestinal mucosa and in the liver and little is available to produce a pharmacological effect. In the treatment of asthma it is either given sublingually (where it escapes the portal circulation) or by aerosol inhaler. Even when given by the latter route about 80 per cent of the administered dose enters the mouth, is swallowed and thus metabolised.

D **TRUE** Tetracycline absorption in the gastrointestinal tract is impaired by the presence of metal cations (Ca^{++}, Mg^{++}, Fe^{++} and Al^{+++}) due to production of in-

27

soluble chelates. Milk which contains large amounts of Ca^{++} should not be taken with tetracyclines.

E TRUE The absorption of griseofulvin is considerably enhanced in the presence of fat, which by stimulating bile secretion appears to enhance dissolution of this poorly water soluble drug (see graph).

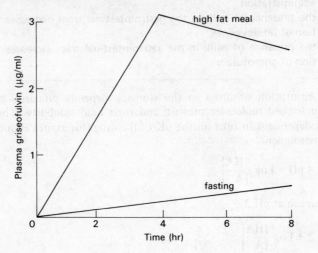

13 Which of the following is/are true

    A probenecid will reduce penetration of penicillin into the cns
    B increasing the fat/water coefficient of a drug increases its rate of entry
        into the cns
    C sulphonamides have greater affinity for plasma proteins than bilirubin
    D warfarin has greater affinity for plasma protein than aspirin
    E globulins are the main protein involved in plasma binding of drugs

---

A FALSE Penicillin is an acid and is actively secreted from the brain by the same mechanism that protects the brain from naturally occurring strong acids and organic ions. The mechanism is similar to that by which penicillin is actively excreted from the proximal tubules of the kidney. Probenecid is a competitive inhibitor at both sites and will therefore facilitate entry of penicillin into the brain, as well as increasing the blood levels.

B TRUE Penetration of a drug into the brain is dependent primarily on its solubility in lipid; a higher fat/water partition coefficient being associated with a higher rate of entry. This is best seen in relation to the rate of appearance of various barbiturates into the cerebrospinal fluid.

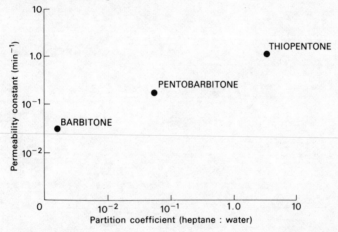

C TRUE Certain groups of drugs bind to a limited number of common binding sites on plasma albumin (see E), and each drug will bind to a degree depending on its concentration in the plasma and its relative binding affinity with the protein. A drug already bound may thus be displaced by a second drug which has a higher binding affinity. Bilirubin is normally transported in the body by plasma albumin and in the presence of sulphonamides will be displaced to cause hyperbilirubinaemia and perhaps jaundice. Administration of sulphonamides is particularly dangerous in the newborn where due to immaturity jaundice may occur anyway; and the high levels of bilirubin can produce permanent damage to the brain.

D FALSE Warfarin in the plasma is about 98 per cent bound to albumin and only a small decrease in binding to 96 per cent doubles the effective plasma concentration. This is equivalent to doubling the dose of warfarin. Such displacement is readily induced by aspirin which may therefore cause bleeding.

E FALSE Albumin is the main protein involved in the plasma binding of drugs, and at least two binding sites on the molecular structure are involved. The first on the N-terminal amino acid (aspartate) is numerically the most important, and binds acid compounds such as fatty acids, salicylates, hormones, bilirubin etc. The second site is to − SH groups and provides a more stable binding, e.g. with disulfiram.

14 Which of the following drugs is/are made more active by metabolism

A senna
B procaine
C levodopa
D cortisone
E thiopentone

A TRUE The glycosides present in senna must be hydrolysed in the small intestine to liberate the anthraquinone purgative. These then either pass through the intestinal lumen or are absorbed into the bloodstream to act on the large intestine.

B FALSE Procaine is an ester of para-amino-benzoic acid (PABA) and in the body is rapidly inactivated by cholinesterase to PABA.

$$H_2N \text{—} \bigcirc \text{—} COOCH_2CH_2 \text{—} N \begin{matrix} /C_2H_5 \\ \backslash C_2H_5 \end{matrix} + H_2O \longrightarrow H_2N \text{—} \bigcirc \text{—} COOH + HO\ CH_2CH_2N \begin{matrix} /C_2H_5 \\ \backslash C_2H_5 \end{matrix}$$

procaine   PABA   diethyl-amino-ethanol

C TRUE Levodopa is a precursor in the synthesis of dopamine. It is used in the treatment of Parkinsonism, a disease in which brain dopamine levels are deficient. Dopamine is not used, because it will not cross the blood/brain barrier, but levodopa is rapidly converted to the inhibitory transmitter dopamine by the enzyme dopa decarboxylase.

D TRUE Cortisone is a relatively ineffective anti-inflammatory agent, but it may be used clinically for this purpose because it is rapidly converted to cortisol (hydrocortisone) by a dehydrogenase enzyme in the liver. Experimental studies in animals have shown that while cortisol has only one and a half times more mineralocorticoid and glucocorticoid activity than cortisone, it is some 700 times more potent as an anti-inflammatory agent.

E FALSE When injected intravenously thiopentone is rapidly taken up into the brain to produce an almost immediate anaesthetic action. This is an action of the parent compound and metabolism (which occurs in the liver) serves only to inactivate it.

15 Conjugation of drugs

A occurs primarily in the liver
B increases their water solubility
C is brought about by microsomal enzymes
D can occur with glycine
E can occur with glucuronic acid

A TRUE Conjugation is a physiological process by which bile salts, bile pigments, various hormones and some drugs are inactivated by addition of another molecule, e.g. glucuronic acid. It occurs mainly in the liver and to a lesser extent in the kidney and lungs.

B TRUE Formation of a conjugate generally makes the drug more polar, which reduces its lipid solubility and increases its water solubility. This in turn means that it is more readily excreted in both urine and bile.

C TRUE Most conjugation reactions are brought about by the non-microsomal enzyme systems. However, a single but nevertheless important synthetic reaction, namely glucuronide formation, is brought about by the microsomal system. As with other microsomal enzymes this reaction may be stimulated following treatment with certain drugs, e.g. phenobarbitone.

D TRUE In humans the amino acids glycine and glutamine serve as conjugating agents, but only with compounds containing a carboxyl group, e.g. salicylic acid. The resulting conjugates are excreted primarily in the urine.

E TRUE The most important conjugation reaction is with glucuronic acid, which unlike the other conjugation reactions is brought about by microsomal enzymes (see C). Important drugs that form glucuronides include aspirin, morphine, chloramphenicol and carbenoxolone.

16 Conjugation of drugs with glucuronic acid to form glucuronides

    A is enhanced in the newborn
    B results in substances with greater fat solubility
    C leads to prolongation of drug action
    D leads to more rapid urinary excretion
    E leads to less rapid biliary secretion

A FALSE Cytochrome P_{450} and glucuronidating systems are generally at a low level of activity at birth and do not reach adult activity for many weeks. In premature babies the levels are particularly low. The inability to conjugate bilirubin and thus prevent its penetration into the cns in part explains the danger of jaundice in the newborn.

B FALSE Conjugation is a synthetic process in which, in this case, glucuronic acid is added to a drug or naturally occuring substance. The resulting molecule is more polar and therefore less soluble in lipid but more soluble in water.

C FALSE In addition to altering polarity of the molecule which might prevent its access to the receptor sites, conjugation may also mask the active group of the drug and effectively detoxify it.

D TRUE Because of its greater solubility in water than the parent compound the glucuronide readily passes into the tubular lumen at the glomerulus to be excreted in the urine. Its poor lipid solubility prevents any significant reabsorption in the kidney tubules.

E FALSE Un-metabolised drugs are not readily secreted in the bile and most drugs that appear there are in a conjugated form, e.g. with glucuronic acid. Once in the intestine, bacterial enzymes may release the free drug which then appears in the faeces. However, this is not the only possibility, and lipid soluble agents may be reabsorbed to undergo further metabolism. If conjugation takes place then biliary secretion will occur again. This cycle is known as the enterohepatic circulation.

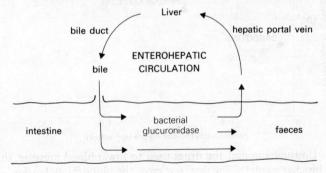

17 Which of the following drugs readily cross the blood/brain barrier

A penicillin G
B hexamethonium
C thiopentone
D guanethidine
E hyoscine

Note: Drugs present in the blood may enter the brain directly or by way of the cerebrospinal fluid (csf). Lipid soluble drugs cross the cerebral capillary walls readily, water soluble molecules cross only slowly and ionised molecules may not enter the brain at all; in fact the choroid plexus actively secretes organic ions from the csf to the blood by a mechanism similar to that operating in the proximal tubule of the kidney.

A FALSE Very little penicillin passes into the csf unless the meninges are inflamed, and then the amount entering is unpredictable. The secretory mechanism of the choroid plexus is largely responsible for maintaining such a low brain level (see Note).

B FALSE Hexamethonium is a highly polar molecule that crosses membranes throughout the body only with difficulty — a fact that explains its poor oral absorption. Its penetration into the brain is therefore poor, but the concentration is kept even lower by active secretion from the choroid plexus (see Note).

C TRUE Thiopentone has a high lipid/water partition coefficient and enters the brain very rapidly to induce general anaesthesia. The higher the lipid/water partition coefficient of a drug the more readily it enters the brain.

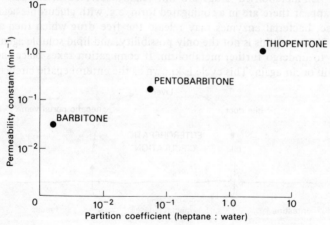

D FALSE Unusual amongst the drugs used to lower blood pressure, the adrenergic neurone blocker guanethidine does *not* cross the blood/brain barrier.

E TRUE Hyoscine is a blocker of the muscarinic actions of acetylcholine. It readily crosses the cns to produce sedation, amnesia, and a useful suppression of motion sickness.

18 Which of the following undesirable reactions to drugs, occuring in a proportion of the population, are due to biochemical defects inherited in a simple Mendelian fashion

    A anaphylactic shock to penicillin
    B agranulocytosis with phenylbutazone
    C raised intraocular pressure following steroid eyedrops
    D reduced action of isoniazid
    E sensitisation of the myocardium with halothane

A FALSE Anaphylactic shock is an acquired defect that may follow a second exposure to a drug molecule, or other antigen. It is described as a Type I hypersensitivity reaction and involves formation of IgE (reaginic) antibody on the surface of mast cells so that following a second antigen exposure, degranulation of the mast cell occurs. This liberates histamine and other autacoids into the circulation to produce the respiratory and cardiovascular effects known as anaphylaxis.

B FALSE Agranulocytosis is a sudden disappearance of granulocytes from the blood which may lead to infective illness. It is a toxic manifestation of therapy with phenylbutazone and deaths can occur as a result (between 2 to 6/100,000 prescriptions). The mechanism is thought to have an immune basis.

C TRUE A rise in intraocular pressure (glaucoma) is generally due to reduced drainage of aqueous humour by the canal of Schlemm, and in susceptible individuals steroids are thought to impair drainage and therefore cause glaucoma. Application of steroids to the eye (for the treatment of inflammatory conditions) may produce one of three effects. In some patients it raises intraocular pressure considerably, in some patients it has no effect, whilst in others it has an intermediate effect. This is a genetically linked phenomenon relating to the presence or absence of two genes determining either an increase in intraocular pressure or no increase in intraocular pressure. The presence of two genes of one type will give either a large effect or no effect whilst one of each produces an intermediate action.

D TRUE The antituberculous drug isoniazid undergoes acetylation in the body by the hepatic enzyme acetyltransferase. The activity of this enzyme is genetically linked and the population shows a bimodal distribution into *slow* and *fast* deactivators. About 50 per cent of Caucasians and Negroes and 90 per cent of Japanese and Eskimoes are fast deactivators, and in these individuals both the pharmacological and toxic actions of the drug are reduced.

E FALSE Halothane, like other fluorinated hydrocarbons, sensitises the myocardium to the β-stimulant effects of catecholamines. It may occur in any patient, but appropriate premedication generally ensures that circulating amine levels are low and that the risk is small. Patients with heart conditions where such cardiac stimulation might be especially dangerous may be protected by giving a β-blocker.

19 The excretion rate of salicylates in the urine will tend to increase following

    A administration of sodium bicarbonate
    B administration of ammonium chloride
    C administration of probenecid
    D lowered plasma albumin levels
    E polyuria

Note: Normally free salicylate in the plasma passes into the filtrate at the glomerules (1) and on into the kidney tubules. Further salicylate is secreted into the urine in the proximal tubules (2) and depending on the pH some is reabsorbed in the distal tubules (3). Acetylsalicylic acid has a pK of 3.5 and in normal acid urine is unionised, so that significant reabsorption will occur.

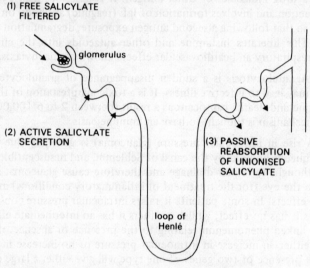

(1) FREE SALICYLATE FILTERED

glomerulus

(2) ACTIVE SALICYLATE SECRETION

(3) PASSIVE REABSORPTION OF UNIONISED SALICYLATE

loop of Henlé

A TRUE By creating an alkaline urine, sodium bicarbonate will increase the degree of ionisation of salicylates in the kidney tubules, impeding passive reabsorption and thus enhancing excretion.

B FALSE Ammonium chloride by creating an acid urine will ensure that salicylates are in the unionised state. Depending on the original pH, excretion will either be unchanged or reduced.

C FALSE Probenecid will compete with salicylates for the transport system in the proximal tubules, thus reducing urinary excretion of the latter.

D TRUE A reduction in circulating albumin will increase the proportion of free salicylate in the plasma and thus the amount entering the tubules. This will increase the amount excreted.

E TRUE A high urine flow impairs passive reabsorption so that more salicylate is lost in the urine.

20 Excretion of

    A aspirin is increased by administration of ammonium chloride
    B penicillin is reduced by administration of probenecid
    C volatile anaesthetics is primarily through the lungs
    D thiopentone explains the rapid recovery from this drug
    E carbenoxolone is primarily in the faeces

A FALSE Aspirin and its metabolites not bound to circulating plasma protein will, at the glomerulus, pass into the kidney tubules. Depending on the degree of ionisation, some of the salicylate will be reabsorbed in the distal tubule. Salicyclic and acetylsalicylic acid are weak acids with a pK of around 4 and at normal acid urinary pH are unionised, so significant reabsorption occurs. By ensuring an acid pH ammonium chloride will either reduce, or have little effect on, aspirin excretion.

B TRUE Penicillin is an acid and is secreted into the proximal tubules of the kidney by the system that is used to excrete phosphoric and sulphuric acid from the body. There is competition for the transport mechanism between the various substances excreted by this route, and probenecid is secreted in preference. This will maintain the blood concentration of penicillin at a higher level for a longer period.

C TRUE Volatile anaesthetics are not only absorbed through the lungs but are also excreted to a major extent by this route. The process is analogous to steam distillation, the greater the vapour pressure of the agent at body temperature the more that will escape in the expired air.

D FALSE Thiopentone is a highly lipid soluble drug which is readily taken up into brain tissue to produce anaesthesia. It equilibrates in the fat of the brain initially, simply because a large proportion of the cardiac output supplies the brain. However, it is also taken up into adipose tissue throughout the body and once the blood concentration falls below that in the brain, thiopentone will leak back into the circulation to be taken up into fat tissue elsewhere. This explains the rapid recovery from thiopentone. Metabolism and excretion occur more slowly as the drug becomes redistributed throughout the body.

E TRUE Carbenoxolone sodium is absorbed primarily in the stomach and excreted mainly in the faeces (about 70 to 80 per cent) via the bile. Some entero-hepatic recirculation occurs and conjugated metabolites appear in the bile.

Pharmacokinetics: related questions 165, 206

21 Which of the following by an action *directly on various enzyme systems* **will greatly modify the rate of metabolism of other drugs**

    A phenobarbitone
    B aspirin
    C amylobarbitone
    D phenelzine
    E imipramine

A TRUE Phenobarbitone when administered regularly for a period of time induces the liver to produce greater amounts of microsomal enzymes. This has two effects; first, it increases the metabolism of the barbiturate so that tolerance develops, and secondly, it increases the rate of metabolism of other substances broken down by the same enzyme system. Drugs affected in this way include warfarin, imipramine and prednisone.

B FALSE Aspirin may dramatically increase the pharmacological and toxic actions of a variety of drugs viz. warfarin, methotrexate, tolbutamide, phenytoin, but it does so by displacing them from their binding sites on circulating plasma protein, not by an effect on metabolising enzymes.

C TRUE Amylobarbitone, in common with other barbiturates, induces liver microsomal enzymes (see A).

D TRUE In addition to inhibiting monoamine oxidase throughout the body phenelzine also inhibits a number of other enzymes, including liver microsomal enzymes. Thus, not only are the actions of amines like amphetamine and phenylephrine affected, but also other drugs such as pethidine and barbiturates.

E FALSE Imipramine is a tricyclic antidepressant that produces interactions with a number of drugs including monoamine oxidase inhibitors and guanethidine. Such effects are not due to alterations in metabolic enzymes, but are pharmacodynamic effects in which the *action* of the drug is modified.

22 Which of the following food substances should be avoided during treatment with monoamine oxidase inhibitors (MAOIs)

    A yoghourt
    B milk
    C broad beans
    D yeast extract
    E Chianti

Note: Amines notably tyramine, present in a range of foods are normally inactivated by mono-amine oxidase (MAO) present both in the lining of the gastrointestinal tract and in the liver. They are consequently without noticeable pharmacological effect. In patients treated with MAOIs the amines are free to enter the circulation where they can bring about release of nor-adrenaline from sympathetic nerves (i.e. they are indirectly acting amines). This will cause massive vasoconstriction and a rise in blood pressure, perhaps in excess of 200 mmHg. This may be sufficient to induce a violent headache and if the pressure rises further may precipitate cerebral haemorrhage. It is known as the 'cheese reaction' because it is provoked most readily by the large amounts of tyramine in cheese.

A TRUE Compared with cheese which may contain 1 mg/g of tyramine, yog-hourt only contains a small amount (<0.2 μg/g). However, there are a number of reports of untoward reactions following its consumption. The extent of the reaction is thought to reflect the extent of bacterial fermentation.

B FALSE Only soured milk, in which the protein has been hydrolysed and the amino acid tyrosine decarboxylated to tyramine, will provoke a reaction in patients receiving MAOIs.

C TRUE Hypotensive crises have been reported in patients receiving MAOIs following consumption of broad beans with their pods. This is due to the high content not of tyramine but of dopa, which is decarboxylated in the body to dopa-mine. Instead of being metabolised by MAO the dopamine provokes a widespread sympathetic stimulation.

D TRUE Yeast extracts may contain as much as 1 to 5 mg/g of tyramine and readily induce hypertensive crises.

E TRUE Wines and beers have been shown generally to provoke untoward reactions in patients receiving MAOIs. This is not thought to be due to the alcohol content but rather to the fermented nature of the beverage and its tyramine content. Amongst them, Chianti has one of the highest tyramine contents (25 μg/ml) and most easily induces the reaction.

23 Patients who are receiving monoamine oxidase inhibitors (MAOIs) of the hydrazine type may produce a more marked response than normal following administration of

    A direct acting amines like noradrenaline
    B mixed acting amines like phenylephrine
    C narcotic analgesics like morphine
    D tricyclic antidepressants like imipramine
    E mild analgesics like aspirin

A FALSE Noradrenaline produces its effect by direct stimulation of receptors, its pharmacological action being curtailed primarily by re-uptake into the sympathetic nerve endings (Uptake 1). Inhibition of monoamine oxidase (MAO) would not thus be expected to affect the action of noradrenaline and experimental observations support this suggestion.

B TRUE Although phenylephrine mainly stimulates receptors by a direct action, it also releases noradrenaline from intraneuronal stores. In the presence of MAOIs the stores of noradrenaline in the nerve are much greater than normal and a much larger quantity of noradrenaline is thus released. Phenylephrine is found in proprietary cold preparations, and its consumption by patients receiving MAOIs may cause a potentially dangerous hypertension.

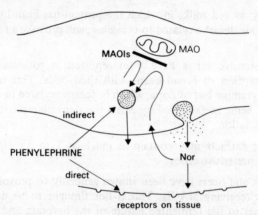

receptors on tissue

C TRUE In some, but not all, patients receiving MAOIs, injection of morphine will provoke a reaction in which the depressant effects of morphine are potentiated. Since respiratory failure, hypotension and coma may result it is recommended that morphine is contraindicated unless a sensitivity test is first carried out. The reaction is in part due to inhibition of liver microsomal enzymes by the MAOI with consequent inhibition of the morphine metabolism.

D TRUE Tricyclic antidepressants are effective antidepressants by virtue of their ability to block the re-uptake of noradrenaline into sympathetic nerves (Uptake 1), thus increasing the amount available to produce an action on the receptor. In patients receiving MAOIs the stores of intraneuronal noradrenaline are much greater than normal, and the amount released following nerve stimulation is also greater; again producing greater receptor action. When these drugs are given together both actions are apparent, and combined therapy of this type has been used to treat depression. However, many severe toxic reactions have been reported including hypertensive crises.

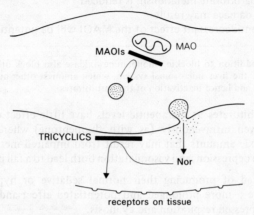

E FALSE There is no evidence that aspirin has a more marked action in the presence of MAOIs.

24 In patients taking monoamine oxidase inhibitors (MAOIs) a single administration of barbiturate may be dangerous because

    A the blood pressure is elevated
    B coma may be produced
    C the barbiturate metabolism is reduced
    D liver damage may result
    E the antidepressant effect of the MAOI will be potentiated

---

Note: MAOIs in addition to blocking monoamine oxidase also block other oxidase enzymes, especially those of the liver microsomal system, which amongst other actions are responsible for the metabolism and hence inactivation of the barbiturates.

A FALSE Barbiturates at therapeutic levels have little effect on blood pressure, except when given intravenously (as with thiopentone) where a slight fall may occur. In the toxic amounts that may result from impaired metabolism or in overdose, myocardial depression, and vasodilatation both lead to a fall in blood pressure.

B TRUE Instead of producing their normal sedative or hypnotic actions the barbiturates have a more prolonged and potentiated effect and coma may occur, with severely depressed respiration and cyanosis.

C TRUE See Note and B.

D FALSE Some MAOIs are hepatotoxic and acute liver damage may occur particularly with the hydrazine group of drugs, e.g. phenelzine, iproniazid. However, although all barbiturates are metabolised to some extent by the liver, there is no evidence that accumulation of unmetabolised barbiturate increases the incidence of hepatocellular damage.

E FALSE A single administration of barbiturate will not significantly modify enzyme levels in the liver, and will not interfere with the metabolism or action of MAOIs. Prolonged administration, by causing enzyme induction, may reduce their efficacy.

25 Aspirin when given to patients receiving other drugs may cause which of the following interactions

    A antagonism of the effect of oral hypoglycaemic agents such as tolbutamide
    B potentiation of the hypotensive action of guanethidine
    C potentiation of the levels of free warfarin in the blood
    D agranulocytosis in a patient taking methotrexate
    E inhibition of the uricosuric action of sulphinpyrazone

A FALSE Aspirin has two actions which will tend to increase the degree of hypoglycaemia, i.e. potentiate the effect of the antidiabetic drug. First, salicylates will displace tolbutamide from its binding site on plasma protein and thus increase its pharmacological effects. Secondly, aspirin may in diabetics have an apparent insulin-like action probably due to increased peripheral utilisation of glucose.

B FALSE The hypotensive action of guanethidine does not appear to be affected by aspirin treatment.

C TRUE About 98 per cent of warfarin in the plasma is bound to albumin, and only a small reduction of the binding capacity to say 96 per cent effectively doubles the free pharmacologically-active concentration. Aspirin binds readily to the same binding sites as warfarin and displaces it into the plasma. The result is a much increased clotting time and the possibility of serious haemorrhage.

D TRUE Like warfarin, methotrexate is bound to circulating plasma protein, and its displacement by aspirin increases the pharmacological effect. This not only means increased killing of malignant cells but also destruction of other rapidly dividing cells, and in particular cells of the bone marrow; so that a sudden reduction of circulating neutrophils occurs, i.e. agranulocytosis.

E TRUE Uric acid is filtered by the glomerulus and totally reabsorbed in the proximal tubules; only that which is subsequently secreted into the distal tubules is normally excreted. Sulphinpyrazone inhibits the proximal tubule mechanism and thus increases uric acid excretion. Aspirin antagonises the uricosuric action of sulphinpyrazone at this site by competing for the secretory mechanism.

26 Which of the following drugs have enzyme-inducing properties

A morphine
B diazepam
C phenytoin
D isoniazid
E amylobarbitone

Note: Enzyme induction refers to the ability of drugs and other chemicals to stimulate the synthesis of drug metabolising enzymes. It is characterised by increased liver weight following hypertrophy of the smooth endoplasmic reticulum and increased production of microsomal protein and cytochrome P_{450}. A number of chemically dissimilar agents have this ability which, in addition to stimulating their own metabolism, also increases the biotransformation of a range of other drugs.

A FALSE The major pathway for the detoxification of morphine is conjugation with glucuronic acid by the non-microsomal enzymes of the liver. Although tolerance will follow its repeated use this is thought to reflect alterations in the pharmacodynamics of morphine (e.g. changes in enkephalin levels) rather than a change in pharmacokinetics, i.e. enzyme induction.

B FALSE Although to some extent metabolised by the microsomal system, diazepam does not induce enzymes. The main pathway of inactivation is conjugation with glucuronic acid. However, there is some evidence that in the presence of other inducers its metabolism is increased.

C TRUE In man phenytoin is largely metabolised by the liver microsomal enzyme system and its metabolism is susceptible to inducers and inhibitors. It is itself only a weak enzyme inducer, but this may be sufficient to reduce the efficacy of both endogenous and administered corticosteroids.

D FALSE Isoniazid is an antituberculous agent which, despite its toxicity, e.g. peripheral neuritis, hepatitis, and the high incidence of resistance, still provides an important therapy. It is an inhibitor of oxidase enzymes throughout the body, especially monoamine oxidase, an action which gives it mild antidepressant properties. It does not, however, induce enzymes.

E TRUE Although phenobarbitone is generally used as the example, all barbiturates metabolised by the liver produce a non-specific enzyme induction, and amylobarbitone is no exception. Several days treatment are required before the effects become apparent.

27 Enzyme induction by barbiturates means that

A more drug metabolising enzyme is present in the liver
B a more active type of enzyme is present in the liver
C barbiturates are destroyed more readily
D warfarin is destroyed more rapidly
E tolerance to barbiturates develops

A TRUE Induction of enzymes following prolonged drug administration means that more enzyme is synthesised by the liver. It is characterised by hypertrophy of the smooth endoplasmic reticulum (the site associated with drug metabolism), increased production of microsomal protein and of cytochrome P_{450}, and by increased liver weight.

B FALSE The additional enzyme synthesised as a result of drug exposure (see A) has similar activity to that normally present.

C TRUE Barbiturates are the substrate for the enzymes which they induce, and so are more readily destroyed and have a reduced pharmacological effect (see also E).

D TRUE The coumarin anticoagulant warfarin is metabolised in the liver by the same enzyme system responsible for barbiturate metabolism. Following enzyme induction, warfarin metabolism is increased and its pharmacological effect reduced.

E TRUE Tolerance or tachyphylaxis may be described as diminished pharmacological response to repeated administration of the same dose of a drug. It may be due to reduced receptor response to the same drug concentration, or as is the case with barbiturates, due to a reduction in the circulating level of drug because of more rapid metabolism.

28 If warfarin is given to a patient who has been habitually taking a barbiturate hypnotic

    A the barbiturate dose will have to be increased to produce the same effect

    B the warfarin will have to be given in bigger than usual doses

    C the patient will bleed excessively following trivial injury

    D the barbiturate has a greater action because it is displaced from binding sites on circulating plasma protein

    E the rate of metabolism of warfarin is slower than normal

---

Note: Prolonged administration of barbiturates induces increased production of liver microsomal enzymes. This not only results in more rapid metabolism of the barbiturate, but also of other substances normally metabolised by these enzymes.

A FALSE Whilst it is true that after enzyme induction, barbiturates will have a reduced pharmacological effect and more must be given to produce the same action, administration of warfarin does not alter the efficacy of the barbiturates.

B TRUE Since warfarin is metabolised by the liver microsomal enzyme system, a dose that in a normal patient would be sufficient to produce the required degree of anticoagulant action, will, in a subject with induced enzymes, be metabolised more quickly and have a reduced action. To achieve the desired pharmacological effect, warfarin would then need to be given in larger amounts.

C FALSE Because warfarin has reduced efficacy (see B) the anticoagulant action of warfarin will be less readily achieved and clotting may occur.

D FALSE About half of a dose of a hypnotic barbiturate (like pentobarbitone) will become bound to protein throughout the body, a factor which extends complete inactivation and excretion over several days. However, the amount bound to plasma albumin is small — perhaps as little as 5 per cent of the administered dose — so that displacement from binding sites will have little effect on the pharmacological action. Warfarin in any case does not appear to displace barbiturates.

E FALSE See B.

Drug Interactions: related questions 127, 165, 168, 170, 220, 238

29 Body weight gain may occur following the clinical use of which of the following drugs

  A carbenoxolone
  B combined progesterone/oestrogen contraceptives
  C thyroxine (in the treatment of adult hypothyroidism)
  D bendrofluazide
  E fenfluramine

A TRUE Carbenoxolone is the disodium salt of the liquorice derivative glycyrrhetinic acid. It has a structure similar to the corticosteroids and is used clinically to treat peptic ulcer. A common side effect is weight gain due to sodium retention and oedema. It is a result of the aldosterone-like action of carbenoxolone.

B TRUE A well recognised side effect of the combined contraceptive pill is body weight gain and women commonly gain up to 1 kg in weight. It is due to salt and water retention caused by the oestrogen component of the pill.

C FALSE Adult hypothyroidism or myxoedema is characterised amongst other features by increasing body weight and oedematous appearance due to the subcutaneous accumulation of a viscid muscinous material. It is due to inadequate output of thyroid hormone. Treatment with thyroxine readily reverses these changes and body weight returns to normal.

D FALSE The thiazide diuretic, bendrofluazide, increases the excretion of sodium and water, the immediate effect of which is a dramatic fall in body weight.

E FALSE Fenfluramine is a trifluoromethyl derivative of phenylethylamine and belongs to the same group of compounds as the more widely known drug, amphetamine. Both substances depress the appetite, but fenfluramine does not possess the powerful cns stimulant actions of amphetamine, and is used in conjunction with dietary control to treat obesity. The effect wears off after a few weeks of treatment.

30 Hypertension is a recognised complication in the use of which of the following groups of drugs

    A tricyclic antidepressants
    B oral contraceptives
    C anti-inflammatory steroids
    D adrenergic neurone blockers
    E β-blockers

A FALSE Tricyclic antidepressants prevent the re-uptake of noradrenaline into adrenergic neurones (Uptake I). This increases the amount of noradrenaline available at the receptor site, and is thought to be the mechanism by which the tricyclics produce their actions on the cns. One might, therefore, expect them to potentiate sympathetic vasoconstriction at the periphery and thus cause hypertension. In practice, however, potentiation of catecholamines on the heart may lead to dysrhythmia and reduced cardiac output, and postural hypotension may occur.

B TRUE Hypertension is a recognised hazard of prolonged use of oral contraceptives, the risk increasing with duration of use. It affects less than 5 per cent of users. The mechanism is unclear but may be due to changes in the renin-angiotensin-aldosterone system.

C TRUE Orally administered anti-inflammatory steroids when taken chronically for the treatment of rheumatoid arthritis commonly disturb the electrolyte balance and this may manifest itself as oedema and hypertension. It is especially likely in patients with renal disease, but all patients receiving prolonged steroid therapy should have their blood pressure checked at regular intervals.

D FALSE Adrenergic neurone blocking drugs (like guanethidine) reduce the release of noradrenaline from sympathetic neurones and thus induce hypotension.

E FALSE β-blockers are useful agents in the treatment of hypertension. Their action is complex and involves reduced cardiac output due to a direct blockade of sympathetic stimuli to the heart, and an overall reduction in sympathetic tone due to an action on the vasomotor centre.

31 Renal damage is a recognised hazard in the use of which of the following drugs

    A penicillamine
    B allopurinol
    C sodium aurothiomalate
    D glyceryl trinitrate
    E daunorubicin

A TRUE Proteinuria may occur during treatment with penicillamine and is probably the result of an immune complex nephritis. If protein loss becomes excessive ($>2g$/day) therapy should be discontinued.

B FALSE Allopurinol is an inhibitor of xanthine oxidase and is used to reduce uric acid production in patients suffering from gout. It causes increased blood levels of xanthine and hypoxanthine which are highly water soluble substances and readily excreted by the kidney. Treatment of gout with agents that increase urinary excretion of uric acid (so-called uricosuric drugs) may on the other hand induce crystalluria and cause renal damage.

C TRUE Between 60 to 90 per cent of an administered dose of gold (given as sodium aurothiomalate) is excreted through the kidney and cumulation occurs in this organ. The effect is to cause damage mainly to the proximal tubules and about 50 per cent of patients receiving crysotherapy show traces of proteinuria at some stage during therapy.

D FALSE Glyceryl trinitrate is rapidly metabolised in the body primarily by the liver to the almost inactive mono and dinitrate. These are excreted in the urine, but renal damage does not occur.

E FALSE Daunorubicin is an antineoplastic antibiotic. In addition to the toxicity characteristic of all cytotoxic drugs, i.e. bone marrow depression, alopecia etc., it is markedly cardiotoxic, but it does not appear to affect the kidney.

32 Which of the following drugs should be avoided or used at reduced dosage in patients who have impaired renal function

    A suxamethonium
    B digoxin
    C d-tubocurarine
    D gentamicin
    E methotrexate

A FALSE The depolarising neuromuscular blocking agent suxamethonium is hydrolysed by pseudocholinesterase in the liver and plasma, initially to succinyl-monocholine and then to succinic acid and choline. Hepatic disease by reducing the availability of enzyme may delay inactivation, but since less than 10 per cent of the drug is excreted unchanged renal disease has little effect on its overall action.

B TRUE Digoxin is eliminated in man, mainly by renal excretion, some 60 to 90 per cent of an administered dose appearing unchanged in the urine. The average plasma half-life is about 36 hours, but in renal disease or in the old (glomerular filtration rate declines with advancing age) this may be prolonged. The nausea and vomiting which can result from digoxin toxicity may be mistakenly ascribed to the uraemia associated with renal failure, and the digoxin overdose may go un-noticed until dangerous arrhythmias occur.

C TRUE Unlike suxamethonium (see A), d-tubocurarine is excreted unchanged in the urine to a significant extent. About one third of an administered dose will appear in the urine over a period of several hours after its injection. In patients with renal insufficiency, its action is prolonged and cumulation may follow multiple doses of the drug.

D TRUE Following parenteral administration gentamicin is almost completely excreted in the urine (by glomerular filtration) and about 70 per cent eliminated within six hours. Although ototoxicity is the most common complication, nephro-toxicity can also occur. In any event, in patients with even mildly impaired renal function the plasma concentration following normal doses will be higher than expected. To avoid toxicity gentamicin must be used with great care and at reduced dosage.

E TRUE Between 40 per cent to 90 per cent (depending on the dose) of metho-trexate is excreted unchanged in the urine. It is both filtered and actively secreted, and extreme caution must be used when administering the drug to patients receiv-ing other drugs secreted by the kidney (with which methotrexate will compete) and to patients with renal insufficiency.

33 Neutropaenia leading to agranulocytosis

A is a feature of chronic corticosteroid therapy
B is a recognised hazard when treating chronic inflammatory conditions with phenylbutazone
C causes resistant bacterial infections in the mouth which should be treated with chloramphenicol
D may occur in patients treated with gold salts
E is *unlikely* to occur in patients treated with vincristine

---

A FALSE Corticosteroids cause lymphocytopaenia due in part to destruction of lymphoid tissue, and in part to redistribution of the lymphocytes in other tissues. This is accompanied by an increased appearance of polymorphonuclear leucocytes in the blood (granulocytosis) due to increased rate of entry from the bone marrow and reduced rate of removal.

B TRUE Of the 1,276 adverse reports on phenylbutazone made to the Committee of Safety on Medicines in the nine years up to 1973 about one third were due to blood disorders, and of these 100 were due to agranulocytosis. There is some evidence that an immune mechanism is involved.

C FALSE Severe necrotising infections especially in the mouth and throat are characteristic of severe neutropaenia and should be treated with non-toxic antibiotics. Chloramphenicol, which in any case should be reserved for use against resistant bacterial strains, is a very toxic drug to the bone marrow. It may cause a dose-related reversible leucopaenia, but fatal aplastic anaemia can also occur.

D TRUE Organic gold salts like sodium aurothiomalate used in the treatment of rheumatoid arthritis are extremely toxic, and reactions occur in about half the patients treated. The most serious are to the bone marrow and include thrombocytopaenia, aplastic anaemia and agranulocytosis, which may prove fatal.

E FALSE Vincristine is a spindle poison. It is used to treat acute leukaemia because of its ability to suppress the formation of leukaemic cells by the bone marrow. Leucopaenia is obviously a hazard of its use.

34 Digitalis toxicity

    A occurs on average in less than 1 per cent of patients treated with the drug
    B occurs less frequently in patients treated with thiazide diuretics
    C can manifest as a gastrointestinal upset
    D can manifest as a fatal arrhythmia without previous warning
    E makes treatment of the patient with isoprenaline hazardous

---

A FALSE Digitalis has a low therapeutic ratio and toxicity occurs in most patients at some stage during their therapy. There is a mortality as a result of toxicity of about 15 per cent, and because it is one of the most commonly prescribed drugs, a large proportion of all drug-induced hospital deaths can be attributed to digitalis.

B FALSE Digitalis is thought to produce its beneficial positive inotropic action by inhibiting the Na^+-K^+ membrane ATPase. The effect of this is to cause intracellular accumulation of Na^+, intracellular depletion of K^+ and a corresponding reduction of transmembrane potential, which in turn increases excitability. By decreasing plasma K^+ levels, thiazide diuretics enhance the loss of K^+ from the cell and hence potentiate digitalis effects, so that toxicity occurs more readily.

C TRUE Anorexia, nausea, and vomiting are among the earliest signs of toxicity; diarrhoea and abdominal pain are common accompanying features in many patients.

D TRUE As digitalis accumulates and signs of toxicity occur, there are changes in the ecg, which indicate increasing cardiac involvement. The PR interval increases, the RS-T voltage is depressed and flattening or inversion of the T wave may occur. Gross conduction defects may ultimately lead to total atrioventricular dissociation, but the alterations in cardiac rate and rhythm are such that almost every type of arrhythmia seen clinically may be initiated. Particularly dangerous is paroxysmal ventricular tachycardia, as a result of increased excitability and automaticity of the ventricles (see E), as this may lead to fatal ventricular fibrillation.

E TRUE Increased myocardial excitability is a feature of digitalis action, and may lead to premature systoles. It is the result of a fall in membrane potential. As toxicity increases, there is commonly an increase in automaticity of pacemaker sites due to the increased rate of spontaneous diastolic depolarisation during phase 4 of the action potential. Isoprenaline has an essentially similar action which by increasing heart rate still further may precipitate ventricular fibrillation.

35 Digoxin toxicity is generally increased in patients who

    A are elderly
    B have impaired renal function
    C are hyperkalaemic
    D have anaemia
    E have liver failure

A TRUE After the age of about 35 years there is a gradual decline in the glomerular filtration rate and in the concentrating capacity of the kidney. The effect is to potentiate and prolong the action of drugs normally eliminated to a significant extent by this route. In the elderly the half-life of digoxin may be increased by as much as 50 per cent over that in the young, and the normal frequency of drug administration would soon lead to toxicity (see also B).

B TRUE Between about 60 to 90 per cent of digoxin is excreted unchanged through the kidney to give a plasma half-life of around 36 hrs. Excretion is by glomerular filtration, and in patients with severe renal failure the plasma half-life may be increased 4 to 5 fold. It is essential in such cases to reduce the frequency of maintenance doses in order to avoid toxicity.

C FALSE Digitalis inhibits the Na^+-K^+ membrane ATPase of cardiac muscle and this is at least part of the mechanism by which it produces its positive inotropic action. The intracellular Na^+ level rises whilst that of K^+ falls. This enhances Ca^{++} release from the sarcolemma which in turn facilitates actin-myosin contraction coupling. In the presence of low extracellular K^+ levels (i.e. hypokalaemia), potassium loss from the cell is accentuated and extrasystoles may occur. This effect is frequently seen when concurrent diuretic therapy increases the excretion of potassium.

D FALSE Anaemia per se does not increase digitalis toxicity although some conditions that cause anaemia, e.g. malnutrition, may independently modify digitalis action, e.g. by causing K^+ depletion.

E FALSE Since digoxin is not extensively metabolised by the liver and depends for its inactivation primarily on urinary excretion (see B), liver failure does not increase its toxicity.

36 Practolol has been withdrawn from general clinical use because it

    A is a non-selective β-blocker
    B is dangerous to give it to asthmatics
    C causes sclerosing peritonitis
    D induces thyrotoxicosis
    E causes ocular damage

A FALSE Practolol was one of the first β-blockers to be used clinically that showed selectivity for β_1-adrenoceptors on the heart (see also B).

B FALSE Severe asthmatics achieve a degree of bronchodilatation by reflex activation of the sympathetic system. If non-selective β-blockers like propranolol are given to such patients the β_2-receptors in the lungs are blocked and bronchoconstriction ensues. The main virtue of practolol was its ability to block cardiac β_1-receptors without causing bronchoconstriction.

C TRUE Two of the most serious adverse reactions with practolol, and those to a large extent responsible for its withdrawal were ocular damage (see E) and sclerosing peritonitis. Both are associated with immunological disturbances. The sclerosing peritonitis is unusual in that it may occur many months after therapy has ceased. Fibrous adhesions are present in the abdomen (and sometimes in the thorax) initially impeding normal organ function, but eventually preventing it altogether.

D FALSE A feature of thyrotoxicosis is the increased response that occurs to sympathetic nerve stimulation, and palpitations commonly occur as a result. Use of a β-blocker will help to alleviate this problem and practolol but for its other toxicity would provide a suitable treatment.

E TRUE The ocular damage that was produced by practolol has been described as the 'dry-eye' syndrome because tear secretion is reduced and conjunctivitis occurs. This led to complaints of burning, gritty discomfort and photophobia. Conjunctival scarring and fibrosis also occurred and where corneal lesions were produced the outcome was loss of vision which in severe cases produced blindness. (See also C.)

Drug Toxicity: related questions 18, 69, 126, 156, 175, 180, 184, 200, 219, 225, 250

37 The transmitter substance at

A symphathetic postganglionic nerve endings is usually noradrenaline
B parasympathetic ganglia is acetylcholine
C sympathetic ganglia is nicotine
D parasympathetic postganglionic nerve endings is muscarine
E bronchodilator sympathetic nerves is isoprenaline

Note: The transmitters at nerve endings in the autonomic and motor nervous system are shown in the following diagram:

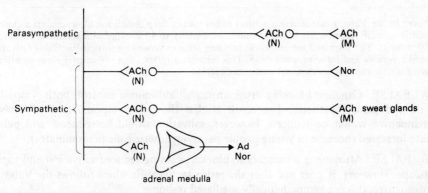

A **TRUE** With the exception of the sweat glands where the transmitter is acetylcholine.

B **TRUE** The transmitter at all ganglia in the autonomic nervous system is acetylcholine.

C **FALSE** The receptors on which the transmitter (acetylcholine) acts at ganglia are described as nicotinic, because nicotine will stimulate them. It is not the transmitter.

D **FALSE** The actions of acetylcholine at all parasympathetic postganglionic nerve endings and at sympathetic nerve endings to the sweat glands are described as muscarinic. This is because the drug muscarine will also stimulate receptors at these sites; it is not the natural transmitter.

E **FALSE** Isoprenaline when administered will produce bronchodilatation. However, it is a synthetic chemical not normally found within the body. The sympathetic nerves to the lungs release noradrenaline.

38 When injected into a young male subject a drug has no effect on resting pulse rate, does not produce a dry mouth, and depresses the increase in heart rate that normally follows the Valsava manoeuvre. The drug

A has ganglion blocking activity
B could be atropine
C could be propranolol
D could be metoprolol
E would be expected to block the tachycardia induced by inhalation of amyl nitrite

---

Note: In the Valsava manoeuvre a subject either takes a deep breath and blows against a closed glottis or more reproducibly blows a column of mercury to 40 mmHg and maintains it there for 10 seconds. The increased intrathoracic pressure reduces venous return, cardiac filling falls and stroke volume and pulse pressure drop. This initiates a reflex from the carotid sinus to effect sympathetic vasoconstriction and cardioacceleration.

A FALSE Ganglion blocking drugs impair all autonomic control, both sympathetic and parasympathetic. The result is that the reflex response to the Valsava manoeuvre would be reduced. However, salivation would be reduced, and pulse rate increased (because in young people parasympathetic tone predominates).

B FALSE Atropine is a muscarinic blocker, causing reduced salivation and vagal escape. However, it does not alter the reflex tachycardia which follows the Valsava manoeuvre; this is a sympathetically mediated response.

C TRUE By blocking β-adrenoceptors propranolol would be expected to prevent the sympathetically mediated increases in heart rate and force of contraction that occur reflexly following the Valsava manoeuvre, but to have no effect on resting heart rate, which in a healthy young adult is primarily under parasympathetic tone. Salivation would not be noticeably affected either, although secretion of amylase (which is under sympathetic β control) may be reduced.

D TRUE Metoprolol is a β_1-selective adrenoceptor blocker but since the cardiac response to exercise is a β_1 effect, the action of this drug is to all intents similar to those of propranolol (see C).

E TRUE Amyl nitrite causes reflex tachycardia following a transient vasodilatation and fall in blood pressure. This reflex is mediated via the sympathetic system, and since a drug producing the features described is a β-blocker (see C), it would be expected to block this tachycardia.

39 Following subcutaneous injection of a clinical dose of a drug into a healthy young adult, dilatation of the pupil and a rise in systolic blood pressure are produced. The drug could be

    A acting by blocking ganglia
    B stimulating β-receptors throughout the body
    C atropine
    D adrenaline
    E morphine

A FALSE Ganglion blocking agents by preventing sympathetic vasoconstriction at the periphery cause a fall in blood pressure; and have little effect on pupil diameter because both dilator (sympathetic) and constrictor (parasympathetic) impulses are equally inhibited.

B FALSE Stimulation of $β_2$-receptors in skeletal muscle would cause vasodilatation and tend to lower blood pressure whilst stimulation of $β_1$-receptors in the heart would cause cardioacceleration and would tend to elevate blood pressure. Such an action is produced by isoprenaline and the resulting effect on systolic blood pressure is variable. β-stimulants would not be expected to dilate the pupil, however: this is an α effect.

C FALSE Atropine by preventing muscarinic stimulation of receptors on the constrictor pupillae produces a dilated pupil. However, by blocking vagal tone which in young adults is high, a tachycardia will generally occur. Blood pressure is little affected and may even fall.

D TRUE Adrenaline has both α and β actions so that it would be expected to dilate the pupil (an α effect). It also increases the heart rate (β action), dilates blood vessels in skeletal muscle (β action) and constricts blood vessels in the skin and splanchnic region (α action). The result of these cardiovascular changes is typically, an increase in systolic blood pressure, a fall in diastolic blood pressure, and a resulting increase in pulse pressure.

E FALSE Morphine characteristically lowers blood pressure (especially on standing) and constricts the pupil. The former is due in part to histamine release from mast cells and in part to central depression of vasomotor tone: the latter is due to stimulation of the IIIrd nerve nucleus so increasing parasympathetic effects on the iris.

40 When given to man a drug causes bradycardia, increased gut motility and pupillary constriction. Which of the following drugs produces this combination of effects

    A histamine
    B morphine
    C acetylcholine
    D noradrenaline
    E neostigmine

A FALSE Histamine causes tachycardia (directly due to stimulation of H_2-receptors on the myocardium and reflexly following peripheral vasodilatation), increased gut motility (direct H_1 effect on longitudinal smooth muscle), but no effect on the pupil.

B FALSE Morphine causes vasodilatation which will have little effect on heart rate in a supine subject, but may cause reflex tachycardia in a standing subject. It also causes gut stasis (and hence constipation) and pin-point pupils (due to stimulation of the IIIrd nerve nucleus).

C TRUE Parasympathetic nerves supply the heart, gut, and pupils, the effects of stimulation being to cause bradycardia, increased intestinal tone and enhanced peristalsis, and contraction of the constrictor pupillae muscles in the iris. Acetylcholine administration would produce similar effects, but because of its rapid metabolism by serum cholinesterase these would be very transient.

D FALSE Noradrenaline, by stimulating α-adrenoceptors in peripheral arterioles, produces a massive increase in peripheral resistance. This causes a rise in mean arterial blood pressure and a reflex bradycardia. However, it relaxes smooth muscle of the gastrointestinal tract and in the eye causes pupillary dilatation.

E TRUE By prolonging and potentiating the effects of acetylcholine released from parasympathetic nerves, neostigmine produces all three effects (see C). With these actions in mind neostigmine is used to slow the heart in paroxysmal tachycardia, postoperatively to improve intestinal tone in paralytic ileus and to improve drainage of aqueous humour by local application to the eye in glaucoma.

41 Hexamethonium

    A blocks both sympathetic and parasympathetic ganglia
    B like decamethonium is a potent blocker at the neuromuscular junction
    C produces peripheral vasodilatation and an increase in skin temperature
    D increases gastrointestinal tone
    E produces a dry mouth

A TRUE Ganglion blocking agents, like hexamethonium, inhibit transmission in both sympathetic and parasympathetic ganglia without selectivity. This inevitably means that a host of side effects accompany the antihypertensive action of these drugs, and consequently limit their usefulness.

B FALSE Both hexamethonium and decamethonium are quaternary ammonium compounds with the common structure $(CH_3)_3 N-(CH_2)_n-N(CH_3)_3$, where n = 6 and n = 10 respectively. Hexamethonium does not cause neuromuscular blockade (see graph), and decamethonium does not have ganglion blocking activity.

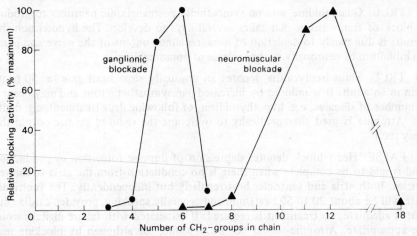

C TRUE By blocking transmission of impulses at sympathetic ganglia in nerve fibres supplying the peripheral arterioles, hexamethonium induces vasodilatation. The outcome of this is a rise in skin temperature, and ultimately therefore a fall in core temperature.

D FALSE The tone of smooth muscle in the gastrointestinal tract is primarily under parasympathetic control. Blocking transmission at the ganglia will *reduce* not increase this tone.

E TRUE Salivary secretion is under autonomic control. Sympathetic activity produces a small amount of thick mucus secretion rich in enzyme content, whilst parasympathetic activity produces a copious watery secretion. Ganglion blockade blocks all secretion, and an unpleasant dry mouth results.

42 Which of the following statements is/are correct

    A pempidine is a useful antihistamine
    B salbutamol produces more tachycardia than isoprenaline
    C guanethidine prevents release of noradrenaline from sympathetic neurones
    D atropine is a rational choice in the treatment of sinus bradycardia
    E atropine is useful in the treatment of complete heart block

A FALSE Pempidine is an orally active ganglion blocking agent.

B FALSE Because isoprenaline produces disturbing and sometimes dangerous tachycardia when it is used as a bronchodilator, experimental investigations into alternatives with greater specificity of action were carried out, salbutamol emerged from these investigations as a drug with a selectivity of action on the lungs. It was largely from this discovery that receptors were divided into two types β_1 (on the heart) and β_2 (on the lungs).

C TRUE Guanethidine acts on sympathetic postganglionic neurones to produce a block of transmission that takes several days to develop. The hypotension that results is due partly to depletion of noradrenaline content of the nerve and partly to inhibition of neuronally evoked release of noradrenaline.

D TRUE Sinus bradycardia denotes an unusually slow heart rate i.e. 50 beats/min in an adult. It is induced by increased parasympathetic tone and may occur in a number of diseases, e.g. hypothyroidism, or following drug treatment, e.g. digitalis. Atropine is used therapeutically to overcome the reduced cardiac output that may result.

E FALSE Heart block denotes depression of impulse formation or conduction, and is said to be complete when there is no conduction from the atria to the ventricles. Both atria and ventricles beat regularly but independently. The ventricular rate will be about 30 to 50 beats/min and generally speaking, provided cardiac output is adequate, no treatment is required. If associated with failure digitalis would be appropriate. Atropine would not be of value, for although by blocking muscarinic receptors at the sinoatrial node it might increase atrial rate, because of the conduction block ventricular rate would be unaffected.

Autonomic Nervous System — General: related questions 3, 5

43 Sympathetic ganglia can be

A blocked by α-methyl dopa
B stimulated by acetylcholine
C stimulated by nicotine
D blocked by pempidine
E stimulated by bradykinin

A FALSE α-methyl dopa acts on noradrenergic neurones where it is converted to α-methyl noradrenaline. Its action is both central on the cardiovascular centre and peripheral on postganglionic sympathetic neurones, and brings about a fall in blood pressure. It has no action directly on ganglia.

B TRUE Acetylcholine is the transmitter substance in ganglia of both the sympathetic and parasympathetic portions of the autonomic nervous system. It causes stimulation of postsynaptic receptors at both sites.

C TRUE Nicotine in low doses will stimulate the so-called nicotinic cholinergic receptors at ganglia (see B). This is seen when a cigarette is smoked.

D TRUE Pempidine is a ganglion blocking agent with the advantage over hexamethonium that it is readily absorbed after oral administration. It is no longer much used for the treatment of hypertension, however, because of the side effects common to all ganglion blocking agents, i.e. postural hypotension, loss of accommodation, constipation, impotence, etc.

E TRUE In relatively high concentrations kinins including bradykinin will stimulate ganglion cells, and cause the release of adrenaline from the adrenal medulla.

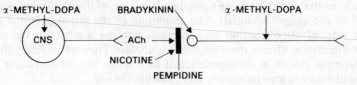

44 The β actions of adrenaline include

A constriction of bronchioles
B increase in the rate of cardiac contraction
C decrease in the force of cardiac contraction
D constriction of arterioles in the skin
E increased glycogenolysis in skeletal muscle

Note: Many of the β effects of adrenaline are thought to be mediated by a rise in the intracellular level of cAMP which by activating different protein kinases brings about the various responses.

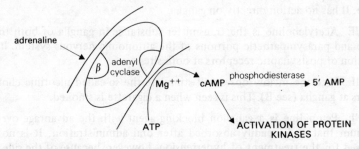

A FALSE The rise in cAMP levels in bronchial smooth muscle causes Ca^{++} to be taken up into stores in the sarcoplasmic reticulum. The Ca^{++} is thus not available for the excitation-contraction coupling mechanism and the bronchioles relax.

B TRUE Adrenaline stimulates β-receptors on the pacemaker cells at the sino-atrial node so that there is a more rapid depolarisation of these cells during diastole (phase 4 of the action potential). The amplitude of the action potential and the maximal rate of depolarisation also increase, but the mechanism by which β-receptor stimulation effects these responses is unclear. They are probably the result of a differential change in the movement of ions across the cell membrane, and an altered availability of ions (especially Ca^{++}) within the cell.

C FALSE The activation of protein kinases by cAMP in cardiac muscle has a number of effects which are thought to be contributory to the positive inotropic action of adrenaline. First, increase in the availability of energy-yielding hexoses occurs because of accelerated breakdown of glycogen (see E). Secondly, phosphorylation of proteins (e.g. troponin) important in contraction may take place, and thirdly, there may be increased availability of Ca^{++}.

D FALSE Constriction of arterioles in the skin is an α not a β effect of adrenaline.

E TRUE The protein kinases activated by β-stimulation (see Note) activate phosphorylase kinase which in turn catalyses the phosphorylation and activation of phosphorylase. This catalyses breakdown of glycogen, but because in muscle glucose-6-phophatase is absent, the end product is lactate.

45 Subcutaneous injection of noradrenaline in man

    A raises systolic blood pressure
    B lowers diastolic blood pressure
    C produces a bradycardia
    D lowers peripheral resistance
    E produces predominantly α actions

A TRUE Systolic blood pressure is primarily dependent on cardiac output, and although noradrenaline causes a bradycardia which might be expected to lower cardiac output and thus systolic pressure, the very considerable increase in peripheral resistance that occurs (see B) swamps this effect and a rise in systolic pressure is typically seen.

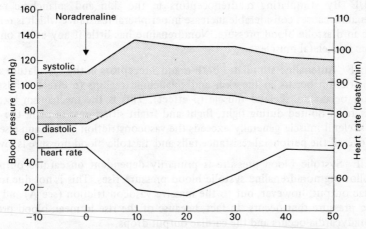

B FALSE By constricting arterioles in the skin and splanchnic regions of the body (see E) noradrenaline produces an increase in peripheral resistance. The rise in diastolic blood pressure reflects this change.

C TRUE Due to the rise in mean blood pressure, baroreceptors in the carotid sinus and elsewhere are stimulated so that reflex vagal slowing of the heart occurs. Any direct action of noradrenaline on β-receptors in the heart will be over-ridden by this bradycardia.

D FALSE See C.

E TRUE The constrictor effect of noradrenaline on the arterioles of the skin and splanchnic area is brought about by stimulation of α-receptors at these sites.

46 Typically when injected into man

    A noradrenaline produces a rise in diastolic pressure due to increased peripheral resistance

    B adrenaline produces a rise in diastolic pressure due to increased peripheral resistance

    C noradrenaline produces a rise in systolic pressure due to increased peripheral resistance

    D isoprenaline produces a rise in diastolic pressure due to increased peripheral resistance

    E tyramine produces a rise in systolic pressure due to noradrenaline release from nerve endings

---

A TRUE By stimulating α-adrenoceptors in the skin and splanchnic regions, noradrenaline causes considerable increase in peripheral resistance which is reflected as a rise in diastolic blood pressure. Noradrenaline has little if any effect on the β-receptors in skeletal muscle.

B FALSE Adrenaline stimulates both α and β-receptors in the vasculature so that vasoconstriction occurs in the skin and splanchnic regions (α effect) whilst vasodilatation occurs in skeletal muscle (β effect). This is the mechanism by which blood is redistributed during fight, flight and fright situations. In man, the dilatation in skeletal muscle generally exceeds the vasoconstriction in skin and elsewhere so that overall the peripheral resistance falls and diastolic blood pressure is lowered.

C TRUE Systolic blood pressure is primarily dependent on cardiac output. In man, following noradrenaline systolic blood pressure rises. This is not due to a rise in cardiac output, however, but to the massive vasoconstriction (see A) and rise in diastolic pressure that occurs. In fact, because of the rise in mean blood pressure, reflex bradycardia occurs and the cardiac output drops.

D FALSE Isoprenaline only stimulates β-receptors causing dilatation in skeletal muscle and an increase in the rate and force of cardiac contraction. Peripheral resistance will, if anything, fall.

E TRUE Tyramine is an indirectly acting amine. It is found in fermented foods like cheese, yeast extract, wine, etc. Normally it is inactivated on ingestion by monoamine oxidase, but if these foods are eaten following treatment with a monoamine oxidase inhibitor or if tyramine is *injected* hypertension will result. The tyramine is taken up into adrenergic neurones and brings about release of noradrenaline at all sympathetic sites throughout the body.

47 Salbutamol

    A is a selective β_1 agonist
    B is useful in the treatment of asthma
    C produces dilatation of blood vessels in skeletal muscle
    D produces accommodation for near vision
    E has its actions competitively antagonised by propranolol

A FALSE Salbutamol selectively stimulates β_2-receptors. This makes it especially useful for treating asthma (see B).

B TRUE Salbutamol is one of the drugs of choice for controlling asthmatic attacks. By stimulating the β-receptors in the lung, it produces dilatation of the bronchioles and inhibition of mast cell degranulation. Furthermore, because of its selective action on β_2-receptors, it less readily causes the unpleasant and potentially dangerous tachycardia seen with non-selective agonists such as isoprenaline.

C TRUE Sympathomimetic amines such as adrenaline when they enter the circulation in large amounts cause vasoconstriction in the skin and splanchnic arterioles (α effect) and dilatation of arterioles in muscle (β effect). This is a physiological mechanism for the redistribution of blood in stress situations. The receptors in the muscle have been classified as β_2 because selective agonists such as salbutamol produce dilatation at this site. This is sometimes seen as a toxic effect during salbutamol use.

D FALSE Accommodation of the lens for near vision is under parasympathetic control and sympathomimetic amines do not modify this process.

E TRUE Propranolol is a competitive antagonist of β-receptor stimulants at all β-receptor sites (both β_1 and β_2) throughout the body.

48 Ephedrine

    A is effective following oral administration
    B is a mixed acting amine, i.e. acts directly on receptors and by causing release of transmitter from sympathetic nerves
    C causes depression of the central nervous system
    D stimulates predominantly α-receptors
    E is contraindicated in patients receiving monoamine oxidase inhibitors (MAOIs)

A TRUE Ephedrine is not a catecholamine, and is not destroyed by monoamine oxidase in the gastrointestinal tract and liver, so escaping metabolism following oral administration.

B TRUE By acting primarily on the adrenergic granules ephedrine brings about release of noradrenaline from nerves and both noradrenaline and adrenaline from the adrenal medulla. It also acts directly on receptors and exhibits substantial effects in reserpine-treated animals and man where tissue stores are depleted.

C FALSE The cns effects of ephedrine are similar but considerably less marked than those of the stimulant amphetamine. Some patients experience tremors, anxiety, restlessness, and insomnia and in overdose delusions and hallucinations.

D FALSE Like adrenaline, ephedrine stimulates α and β-receptors. This action is both directly on the receptors and through the release of endogenous transmitter (see B).

E TRUE Following treatment with MAOIs, intraneuronal levels of monoamines increase, so that mixed-acting and indirectly-acting amines will produce a greater than normal effect. Marked and potentially dangerous hypertension can result. The action of ephedrine is similar in this respect to phenylephrine (see diagram Q23B, page 40).

49 β-adrenoceptor blockers are useful in the management of

    A heart failure
    B bronchial asthma
    C angina pectoris
    D intermittent claudication
    E thyrotoxicosis

A FALSE Heart failure is a chronic inability of the ventricles to maintain an adequate output of blood for the needs of the body. It may follow increases in work load on the heart such as valve disease or hypertension, or the changes in cardiac muscle which result from infarction. One of the compensatory features of failure is an increase in adrenergic drive to the heart and a rise in the rate of contraction. β-blockers by reducing the drive will slow the heart and may make the failure worse.

B FALSE Asthma is characterised by severe constriction of the bronchioles, but most sufferers do not feel the full consequences of this because a reflex is brought into play that moderates the constriction; sympathetic nerves supplying the lungs are stimulated and a degree of physiological antagonism is achieved. Administration of a β-blocker will prevent this homeostatic mechanism and an asthmatic attack may be precipitated.

C TRUE In patients who have angina, there is atherosclerotic narrowing of the coronary arteries, so that when the heart rate rises (following excercise or emotional upset) insufficient oxygenated blood perfuses the myocardium. This allows metabolites to build up and ischaemic pain results. β-blockers by preventing the sympathetically-induced increases in heart rate can be used prophylactically to reduce the frequency and severity of attacks.

D FALSE Intermittent claudication is a painful ischaemic spasm usually of the calf muscle that is brought on by walking and may cause the patient to limp. It is due to atherosclerotic narrowing of major arteries supplying the leg. Treatment includes various vasodilator drugs, but β-blockers by reducing cardiac output and by preventing β-receptor-mediated dilatation of arterioles in skeletal muscles may make the condition worse.

E TRUE In hyperthyroidism, the increased secretion of tri-iodothyronine (T_3) and thyroxine (T_4) in addition to raising the metabolic rate, increases the sensitivity of tissues to sympathetic activity. Severely thyrotoxic patients commonly have a raised heart rate and sometimes dysrhythmias occur. β-blockers are useful in controlling these conditions.

AUTONOMIC NERVOUS SYSTEM

50 Propranolol

A is a useful drug in the treatment of hypertension
B will reduce exercise-induced tachycardia
C reduces myocardial oxygen consumption
D has quinidine-like activity
E is a weak local anaesthetic

A TRUE Propranolol is a useful agent in the treatment of mild to moderate hypertension. Its mechanism of action is complex and not altogether clear. By blocking β-receptors it will reduce both the rate and force of cardiac contraction which will in turn reduce systolic blood pressure. However, the clinical effect of propranolol may take as long as 8 weeks to reach full effect, and an action on the cns to reduce overall sympathetic tone seems a more likely explanation. Other possibilities include reduced release of renin by the kidney and thus reduction in circulating angiotensin, and long term adaptation of peripheral resistance to a reduced cardiac output.

B TRUE The increase in heart rate during exercise is brought about by sympathetic nerve stimulation and/or release of adrenaline into the circulation from the adrenal medulla. Since stimulation of β-receptors occurs, propranolol will antagonise the effect.

C TRUE By preventing sympathetically-induced increases in heart rate and force of contraction, propranolol reduces heart work and thus myocardial oxygen consumption.

D TRUE Propranolol and some other β-blocking drugs have important actions directly on cell membranes which are commonly described as membrane stabilising, quinidine-like, or local anaesthetic. The general effect on the myocardium is to slow conduction and to reduce excitability. However, clinically such actions are only seen at toxic doses and do not appear to contribute to the beneficial actions of β-blockers in the treatment of cardiac dysrhythmias.

E TRUE See D.

51 The β-blocker propranolol

A will block the actions on the heart of circulating adrenaline but not those of noradrenaline released from sympathetic nerves

B does not cross the blood/brain barrier

C is useful in the management of phaeochromocytoma

D is a rational choice of treatment in incomplete heart block

E is contraindicated in anxiety states

A FALSE Both adrenaline released from the adrenal medulla and noradrenaline released from sympathetic nerves supplying the heart will stimulate β-receptors to bring about an increase in the rate and force of cardiac contraction. The β actions of both transmitters are antagonised by propranolol.

B FALSE Propranolol readily penetrates into the brain, and this seems to be a prerequisite in the mechanism by which it lowers blood pressure (i.e. central reduction of sympathetic tone). The vivid dreams experienced by some patients are also evidence of a cns action.

C TRUE Phaeochromocytoma is a tumour of the adrenal medulla, responsible for between 0.5 to 1.0 per cent of cases of hypertension. The clinical features of the disease are due to excess secretion of adrenaline and/or noradrenaline into the circulation, and include hypertension and palpitations. The latter and other β stimulant effects can be controlled with propranolol whilst the hypertension and other α effects can be controlled with phenoxybenzamine. Cover should be provided with both drugs during surgical removal of the tumour.

D FALSE In incomplete heart block there is impaired conduction of impulses in the atrioventricular bundle which results in slowing of the rate and in some cases dropped beats. Increase in the stroke volume may compensate for the reduced cardiac output but if hypotension leading to cerebral anoxia is likely, or if the rate falls so that arrest may occur suddenly, treatment to increase the heart rate should be given, e.g. isoprenaline. β-blockers may make matters worse.

E FALSE Anxiety neuroses manifest themselves by emotional disturbances and autonomic nervous system changes. The predominant feature varies widely from one patient to another, but if they are conscious of a forceful or rapidly beating heart then a β-blocker like propranolol may be beneficial.

52 Ergotamine is

A a powerful vasoconstrictor
B useful in the treatment of postpartum haemorrhage
C an α-adrenoceptor blocker
D useful in the treatment of migraine
E a 5-hydroxytryptamine (5-HT) antagonist

A TRUE Ergot alkaloids in general produce complex actions on the cardiovascular system. With ergotamine these include a central reduction in sympathetic tone, a peripheral α-adrenoceptor blocking action (see C), and a powerful peripheral vasoconstriction (which following prolonged or excessive use can lead to vascular insufficiency and gangrene).

B FALSE Although, when given intravenously, ergotamine will induce postpartum contraction of the uterus it has a more delayed onset of action and is more toxic than ergometrine, and is ineffective orally. Ergometrine is used in preference.

C TRUE Ergotamine has a classic place in pharmacology in that it was used by Sir Henry Dale to demonstrate the 'adrenaline reversal phenomenon' in which the pressor (α-vasoconstrictor) action of adrenaline was abolished to reveal the depressor (β-dilator) action. In some tissues ergotamine is thought to be a partial agonist producing initially α-stimulation and hence vasoconstriction (see A) followed by α-blockade.

D TRUE The aetiology of migraine is complex and poorly understood, but ergotamine is a useful, be it all potentially toxic, therapy. It is thought to act by causing vasoconstriction and thus reducing the amplitude of arterial pulsations in the cranial arteries, although α-blockade and anti- 5-HT activity (see E) may also play a role.

E TRUE Ergotamine is chemically related to methysergide, and like it will inhibit the actions of 5-HT. Since both drugs are effective in migraine control, 5-HT may be implicated in the aetiology of the disease.

Autonomic Nervous System — Sympathetic: related questions 36, 73, 103, 169, 172

53 The action of acetylcholine released from nerve terminals is limited by

    A membrane bound enzymes
    B oxidation
    C pseudocholinesterase
    D breakdown to choline
    E neostigmine

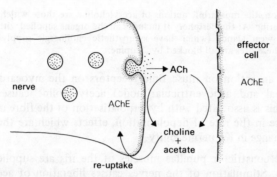

A TRUE The acetylcholinesterase enzymes (see C) responsible for acetylcholine degradation have been shown by histochemical analysis to be associated with both the pre- and postjunctional membranes. It is thought that acetylcholinesterase associated with the nerve membrane protects it from the effects of acetylcholine whilst that on the postjunctional membrane limits the duration and extent of receptor stimulation.

B FALSE Acetylcholine is hydrolysed (not oxidised) to choline and acetate.

$$CH_3COOCH_2CH_2N^+\!\!-\!\!CH_3 \xrightarrow[+\ H_2O]{AChE} HOCH_2CH_2N^+\!\!-\!\!CH_3 + CH_3COOH$$

     acetylcholine   choline   acetic acid

C FALSE The membrane bound enzyme is true (acetyl)cholinesterase; pseudo (butyryl)cholinesterase is found in plasma and non-nervous tissue and is not thought to have an important role in controlling the action of acetylcholine at nerve endings.

D TRUE Choline is produced by metabolism of acetylcholine (see B) and about 50 per cent of it is taken back into the nerve to provide a source for the synthesis of fresh acetylcholine.

E FALSE Neostigmine is an anticholinesterase drug and as such will potentiate the extent and duration of action of acetylcholine released from cholinergic neurones.

54 The muscarinic actions of acetylcholine include
A slowing of the heart
B constriction of the pupil
C accommodation of the eye for distant vision
D increased secretions in the gastrointestinal tract
E increased peristalsis

Note: By definition, the muscarinic actions of acetylcholine are those which can be mimicked by the drug muscarine. At the periphery it includes all the organs supplied with parasympathetic nerves, and the sweat glands (which have sympathetic cholinergic supply). The actions of acetylcholine at these sites are all blocked by atropine.

A TRUE By an action on muscarinic receptors on the myocardium (especially at the sinoatrial and atrioventricular node) acetylcholine causes inhibition of cardiac rate. This is associated with hyperpolarisation of the fibre membrane and a marked decrease in the rate of depolarisation, effects which are thought to be due to a selective change in K^+ permeability.

B TRUE The constrictor pupillae muscles of the iris are supplied by parasympathetic nerves. Stimulation of the nerves causes liberation of acetylcholine and constriction of the pupil.

C FALSE The ciliary muscles which control the shape of the lens are indeed supplied by parasympathetic nerves, but stimulation causes the muscles to contract and the lens to bulge, enabling accommodation for *near* (not distant) vision.

D TRUE Parasympathetic nerves supplying the gastrointestinal tract when stimulated bring about secretion at various sites (e.g. acid and pepsin in the stomach). This is a muscarinic effect of the released acetylcholine and is blocked by atropine.

E TRUE The parasympathetic (cholinergic) supply to the gastrointestinal tract can also evoke an increase in tone of the smooth muscle and enhance peristalsis. Advantage is taken of this fact in treating the paralysis of the gut which may follow abdominal surgery, by giving long lasting cholinomimetics (e.g. carbachol).

55 Parasympathetic mimetics and potentiators are useful in the treatment of

    A peptic ulcer
    B Parkinson's disease
    C atony of the bladder following surgery
    D paralytic ileus
    E chronic glaucoma

A FALSE Gastric acid and pepsin secretion may be induced by vagal stimulation, and drugs which have a similar action may aggravate peptic ulceration. Drugs with anticholinergic activity, e.g. propantheline, have some limited action in reducing acid secretion, but there is no consistent evidence that they improve ulcer healing and many would advocate that they should no longer be used.

B FALSE In Parkinson's disease low levels and reduced secretion of the inhibitory transmitter dopamine from nerves in the nigrostriatal pathway mean that cholinergic nerves acting on cell bodies in the same area will have a greater than usual effect. Muscarinic antagonists by blocking the action of acetylcholine may therefore have a beneficial action, but parasympathetic mimetics and potentiators (if they penetrated into the cns) might make things worse.

C TRUE Lack of tone in the bladder wall and flaccid paralysis of the intestine are common sequels to abdominal surgery. Induction of micturition and return to normal gut function can be achieved with drugs of this type.

D TRUE See C.

E TRUE The high intraocular pressure of glaucoma can be relieved by drugs that induce miosis, a manoeuvre which increases the filtration angle through the canal of Schlemm, so allowing improved outflow of aqueous humour from the anterior chamber of the eye. Both mimetics and potentiators of the parasympathetic system have this action.

56 The anticholinesterase, neostigmine

A acts for several days
B provides a substrate for the enzyme
C phosphorylates cholinesterase
D reverses the action of carbachol
E readily crosses the blood/brain barrier

A FALSE A therapeutic dose of neostigmine would be expected to last for several hours only. At least part of the metabolism is due to destruction by cholinesterase (see B).

B TRUE When cholinesterase hydrolyses acetylcholine to choline, the enzyme becomes acetylated, but only for a short period and regeneration of the active enzyme occurs rapidly in the presence of water. Neostigmine like acetylcholine provides a substrate for the enzyme, being partly broken down in the process. However, the enzyme becomes carbamylated, and regeneration of the active enzyme is many million times slower than with the acetylated enzyme (i.e. anticholinesterase activity is demonstrated).

C FALSE The enzyme is carbamylated not phosphorylated (see B).

D FALSE Carbachol is resistant to cholinesterase, and would not therefore have its action modified by an anticholinesterase.

E FALSE Because of its charged quaternary structure, neostigmine passes into the brain only with difficulty.

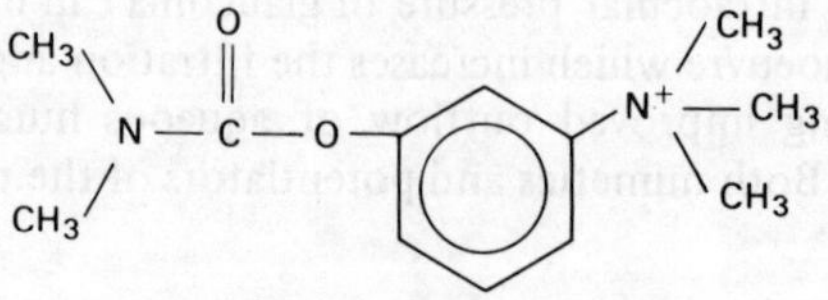

neostigmine

57 Organophosphorus anticholinesterases

A have an irreversible action and therefore have no clinical usefulness
B phosphorylate cholinesterase
C inhibit specific (acetyl)cholinesterase more readily than pseudocholinesterase
D can have their action on the enzyme reversed in the early stages by atropine
E are readily absorbed through the skin

A FALSE The interaction between organophosphorus agents and cholinesterase if allowed to continue is irreversible, and as such excludes the systemic use of these compounds. However, some members of the group, e.g. dyflos, ecothiopate, when administered into the conjunctival sac provide a prolonged miosis which is of value in lowering the raised intraocular pressure of chronic glaucoma.

B TRUE Organophosphorus agents complex with cholinesterase initially in a reversible fashion with the esteratic site of the enzyme. This is rapidly followed by phosphorylation and the formation of an irreversible bond.

C FALSE These substances cause a preferential inhibition of pseudocholinesterase.

D FALSE Although atropine is a recommended treatment for overcoming the effects of anticholinesterase poisoning, it will not interfere with the binding of organophosphorus agents to the cholinesterase enzyme. A useful agent in this respect is pralidoxime which if given soon enough after exposure to the organophosphorus agent will dephosphorylate the enzyme. It must be given before so-called 'ageing' of the phosphorylated enzyme takes place.

E TRUE Substances in this group are easily absorbed through the skin and this provides a serious hazard to agricultural workers who use them as insecticides.

58 Subcutaneous hyoscine injection in a normal subject characteristically produces

    A an increase in heart rate
    B an increased light reflex
    C sedation
    D increased blood pressure
    E sweating

A FALSE Although hyoscine is a competitive antagonist of the muscarinic actions of acetylcholine on the heart, which might be expected to cause an increase in heart rate, it is also a central depressant. By causing both increased vagal firing and by inducing sedation (see C) heart rate tends to fall.

B FALSE The light reflex refers to the ability of the iris to constrict when a light is shone in the eye. As excessive light shines on the retina so the parasympathetic nerves supplying the constrictor pupillae are stimulated. Acetylcholine is then released which stimulates muscarinic receptors to effect pupillary constriction. Hyoscine by blocking the muscarinic receptors will abolish the reflex, and this will occur to some extent even when given by injection.

C TRUE Central depression to cause drowsiness, amnesia, fatigue and even sleep is a feature of hyoscine use. It is of some advantage when hyoscine is given for premedication, but a disadvantage when using it for treating motion sickness.

D FALSE By virtue of the reduced heart rate and sedation a slight fall in blood pressure may accompany use of hyoscine.

E FALSE Sweat glands although anatomically innervated by the sympathetic nervous system are supplied with cholinergic fibres, so that hyoscine will prevent sweating. The effect may be sufficient to raise the body temperature.

59 Subcutaneous atropine injection in healthy young subjects characteristically produces

    A an increase in heart rate
    B an increase in salivation
    C constriction of the pupil (if the dose is adequate)
    D an hypnotic effect
    E accommodation of the lens for near vision

A TRUE As a blocker of the muscarinic actions of acetylcholine, atropine would be expected to reduce vagal tone and thus allow an increase in heart rate. One of the reasons for using atropine as a premedication is its ability to prevent excessive vagal slowing of the heart.

B FALSE Salivation is under both sympathetic and parasympathetic control, the latter causing a copious watery secretion. When atropine is given an unpleasant dry mouth results and secretion following stimuli, e.g. sucking sweets, is much reduced. Reduction of salivary and mucus secretions make it of value for premedication.

C FALSE Atropine (or its derivatives) may be applied directly to the eye to produce mydriasis and thus enable examination of the fundus. When given by injection a similar effect is seen, provided adequate blood levels are achieved.

D FALSE Atropine has an overall stimulant effect on the cns and unlike the related drug hyoscine does not cause hypnosis or sedation.

E FALSE Accommodation of the lens for near vision is brought about by release of acetylcholine from parasympathetic nerves supplying the ciliary muscles. These contract and allow the lens to bulge, so focussing light from near objects onto the retina. Atropine by competing with the acetylcholine will prevent this process, the lens will return to its flattened shape and the eye will focus only on distant objects.

60 Hyoscine

    A is also called scopolamine
    B stimulates the vagus centrally
    C inhibits motion sickness
    D is a ganglion blocking agent
    E reduces mucus secretion

A TRUE The approved name of hyoscine in the USA is scopolamine. It derives from the name of the shrub Scopolia carniolica from which it was originally extracted. Hyoscine is also found in Hyoscyamus niger (henbane). Omnopon and scopolamine is the traditional combination of drugs used for premedication. Omnopon is an extract of opium, the approved name of which is papaveretum.

B TRUE Unlike atropine, hyoscine when given at normal therapeutic doses does not produce an increase in heart rate due to muscarinic blockade of the vagus nerve. Instead a gradual decline in heart rate is seen. This may be ascribed to both stimulation of the vagus centrally, and to the attainment of a basal state due to central depression (see C).

C TRUE Hyoscine is a useful agent for treating vomiting primarily of vestibular origin such as motion sickness and Ménière's disease. Its prolonged use is complicated by the parasympathetic blockade it causes and its central sedative action. The precise site of action is obscure, but most probably involves blockade of cholinergic pathways in the emetic centre and reduction of stimuli from the cortex and vestibular apparatus (see diagram Q140, page 161).

D FALSE Acetylcholine released from preganglionic fibres at the ganglia stimulates nicotinic receptors on the postganglionic fibre to initiate passage of a nerve impulse. Nicotinic receptors are not blocked by muscarinic antagonists such as hyoscine.

E TRUE Mucus secretion in the nasal, respiratory and alimentary tracts is stimulated by acetylcholine released from parasympathetic nerves. This is a muscarinic action and is therefore blocked by hyoscine.

61 Dilatation of the pupil of the eye may be obtained by local administration of

A homatropine
B physostigmine
C cocaine
D salbutamol
E phenylephrine

Note: Sympathetic nerve stimulation induces dilatation by contraction of the radially arranged smooth muscles of the dilator pupillae. Parasympathetic nerve stimulation induces constriction by contraction of the circularly arranged smooth muscles of the constrictor pupillae.

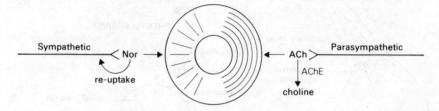

A **TRUE** By blocking parasympathetic muscarinic effects homatropine induces dilatation, although the drug of choice for this purpose in opthalmoscopy is another cholinergic blocker, tropicamide which causes less disturbance of accommodation.

B **FALSE** By preventing the breakdown of acetylcholine, the anticholinesterase physostigmine causes miosis. This leads to improved drainage of aqueous humour through the canal of Schlemm and a reduction of intraocular pressure which may be of value in glaucoma.

C **TRUE** By inhibiting the re-uptake of noradrenaline back into the nerve fibre, cocaine has a potentiating action on sympathetic nerve function and produces pupillary dilatation.

D **FALSE** Salbutamol is a β_2-stimulant which if applied locally to the eye has little if any action on the pupil. It has, however, been used in the eye to treat glaucoma by virtue of its ability to reduce secretion of aqueous humour.

E **TRUE** Predominantly an α-agonist, phenylephrine produces dilatation of the pupil, and is used clinically to facilitate examination of the fundus.

62 If phenylephrine is applied to one eye and atropine to the other eye of a human subject

    A both cause constriction of the pupil
    B only phenylephrine abolishes the corneal reflex
    C neither affect accommodation
    D only atropine causes loss of the light reflex
    E both cause marked vasoconstriction

Note:

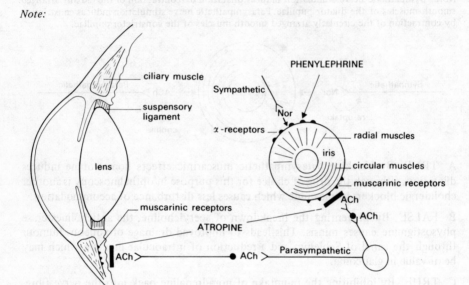

A FALSE Atropine dilates the pupil by blocking the constrictor action of acetylcholine; phenylephrine dilates the pupil by direct stimulation of α-receptors on the dilator pupillae muscle of the iris.

B FALSE The corneal or 'blink' reflex occurs when the surface of the cornea is mildly stimulated by a foreign body (e.g. a wisp of cotton wool). Local anaesthetics by anaesthetising sensory nerves will abolish this reflex but neither phenylephrine nor atropine have this action.

C FALSE Acetylcholine released from parasympathetic nerves supplying the ciliary muscle normally causes contraction; by relaxing the suspensory ligament this allows the lens to bulge for near vision. Atropine thus prevents accommodation.

D TRUE Reflex constriction of the pupil when a light is shone in the eye is effected by contraction of the parasympathetically innervated constrictor pupillae. Thus atropine will abolish the light reflex. Phenylephrine, although producing mydriasis, does not interfere with the reflex pathway; but because it is operating against an opposing set of muscles, constriction may be more sluggish.

E FALSE Vasoconstriction of the conjunctiva is a feature of sympathomimetic substances applied to the eye. Thus cocaine, adrenaline and phenylephrine all show marked blanching of the conjunctiva. Atropine has no significant effect.

63 If applied to the eye

A atropine would cause loss of the light reflex
B procaine would readily cross the mucous membranes to induce corneal anaesthesia
C cocaine would cause vasoconstriction of the conjunctiva
D salbutamol would relieve glaucoma
E castor oil would cause irritation

A TRUE Release of acetylcholine from nerves supplying the constrictor pupillae muscles of the iris is the mechanism by which constriction of the pupil is normally brought about in bright light. Atropine will block the action of acetycholine, thus dilating the pupil and preventing its constriction in response to light. Use of atropine (or its derivatives) in this way enables examination of the retina.

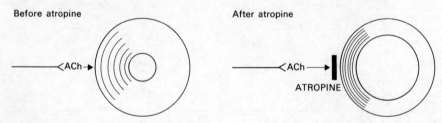

Before atropine   After atropine

B FALSE Procaine does not easily cross mucous membranes and as such would be unsuitable for inducing corneal anaesthesia.

C TRUE By blocking the re-uptake of noradrenaline released from sympathetic nerves supplying blood vessels of the conjunctiva, cocaine potentiates the normal vasoconstrictor tone. Blanching of the conjunctiva normally follows application of cocaine to the eye.

D TRUE Pupillary dilatation following use of sympathomimetic agents in the eye is an α effect, and would be expected to aggravate glaucoma by impeding drainage from the angle of the eye. Salbutamol is a selective β_2-agonist and one would suspect that it is inactive. However, by reducing secretion of aqueous humour β-stimulants produce a limited fall in intraocular pressure.

E FALSE Castor oil is a purgative which following ingestion is hydrolysed by intestinal lipases to glycerol and ricinoleic acid. The latter is a powerful irritant which by contracting the smooth muscle of the small instestine causes purgation. However, when applied to the eye, castor oil is not metabolised in this way and provides a soothing application for allaying irritation due to foreign bodies.

64 If applied directly to the eye
  A cocaine would produce loss of the corneal reflex
  B cocaine would dilate the pupil
  C physostigmine would constrict the pupil
  D physostigmine would impair accommodation for near vision
  E amethocaine would dilate the pupil

A TRUE Cocaine is a local anaesthetic which would anaesthetise the cornea, and thus abolish the normal corneal (blink) reflex.

B TRUE Following release from sympathetic nerves the action of noradrenaline is limited by a process of re-uptake back into the nerve (Uptake 1). Cocaine will block this re-uptake process (see diagram) thus potentiating the action of noradrenaline. The effect in the eye would be to induce contraction of the radial smooth muscles of the pupil, i.e. dilatation would occur.

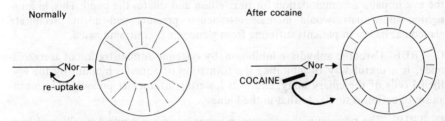

C TRUE The circular smooth muscles of the pupil constrict following stimulation of the parasympathetic nerves which supply it. The acetylcholine which they release has its action limited by cholinesterase present in the junctional gap. Administration of an anticholinesterase like physostigmine inhibits this enzyme so that the action of the acetylcholine is potentiated, and since the pupil is under continuous nervous tone constriction occurs.

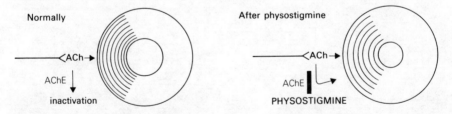

D FALSE Accommodation for near vision is achieved by stimulation of parasympathetic nerves supplying the ciliary muscles. Physostigmine which potentiates parasympathetic effects (see C) would therefore improve accommodation for near vision (i.e. bring the near-point nearer).

E FALSE Amethocaine is a local anaesthetic but it does not possess the ability to potentiate sympathetic nerve activity like cocaine, (see B), and pupil diameter is unaffected.

65 Which of the following drugs would be expected to lower intraocular pressure in glaucoma

   A ecothiopate
   B atropine
   C acetazolamide
   D pilocarpine
   E succinylcholine

A TRUE Ecothiopate is an organophosphorus anticholinesterase which has a powerful miotic action lasting 12 to 24 hours. Constriction of the pupil in this way increases the filtration angle through the canal of Schlemm and thus increases the outflow of aqueous humour from the anterior chamber. The effect is to lower intraocular pressure.

B FALSE Atropine by antagonising the muscarinic actions of acetylcholine in the eye impairs accommodation for near vision and dilates the pupil. This, in long-sighted individuals, would increase intraocular pressure and might precipitate glaucoma. Its use in patients suffering from glaucoma is contraindicated.

C TRUE Carbonic anhydrase inhibition, by systemic administration of acetazola-mide, is a useful way of inhibiting the formation of aqueous humour by the epithelial cells of the ciliary body, and thus lowering intraocular pressure. The mechanism of action is similar to that in the kidney.

D TRUE The parasympathomimetic, pilocarpine, when applied locally will have a similar beneficial miotic action to that seen with the anticholinesterase group of drugs (see A).

E FALSE Succinylcholine is a short acting depolarising neuromuscular blocking agent which would have no effect on the smooth muscle of the iris.

66 d-tubocurarine-induced muscle paralysis

A is caused by prolonged depolarisation of the endplate
B lasts for about five minutes
C is antagonised by neostigmine
D is prolonged when serum cholinesterase activity is low
E is preceded by fasciculations

A FALSE d-tubocurarine is a competitive antagonist of acetylcholine at receptors on the motor endplate, and as such prevents the depolarisation induced by acetylcholine.

B FALSE d-tubocurarine is excreted either unchanged or following metabolism by the liver and a therapeutic dose in man produces a blockade that wears off after 20 to 30 minutes.

C TRUE Because it is a competitive antagonist of acetylcholine the action of d-tubocurarine is overcome when the level of acetylcholine increases. This occurs in the presence of the anticholinesterase neostigmine.

D FALSE Since d-tubocurarine is not metabolised by serum (pseudo) cholinesterase the level does not materially affect the action of d-tubocurarine. Furthermore, the level of acetylcholine at the neuromuscular junction is dependent on local activity of acetyl (true) cholinesterase not on serum cholinesterase.

E FALSE Fasciculations (muscle twitching) are characteristic of the onset of action of depolarising neuromuscular blockers like suxamethonium and are due to the initial depolarisation of the endplate. They are not produced by d-tubocurarine.

67 Curare (d-tubocurarine)-induced neuromuscular blockade

    A is potentiated by ether anaesthesia
    B is accompanied by ganglionic blockade
    C is potentiated in patients suffering from myaesthenia
    D may be accompanied by histamine release
    E paralyses the respiratory muscles first

A TRUE Ether has a weak non-depolarising blocking action at the motor end-plate and will synergise with curare.

B TRUE Curare blocks not only the nicotinic actions of acetylcholine at the neuromuscular junction, but to a lesser extent also those at the ganglia. This may cause hypotension and oozing of blood at the site of operation.

C TRUE Myasthenia gravis is a condition in which there is impaired transmission at the neuromuscular junction. The cause is not clear, but failure of acetylcholine synthesis or release, or insensitivity of the endplate receptors to acetylcholine (perhaps due to a circulating curare-like agent) are all possibilities. Regardless which of these explanations is correct, curare will produce a relatively unopposed action and a greater than normal blockade.

D TRUE d-tubocurarine is a complex quaternary ammonium compound that is capable of releasing histamine from mast cells; locally this may cause itching but systemically the result may be a fall in blood pressure or bronchospasm.

E FALSE The muscles of the face, jaw and throat are the first to be paralysed, and although some loss of respiratory function occurs relatively early, reflex firing down the phrenic and intercostal nerves ensures that respiration ceases only after paralysis of all other muscles.

68 Suxamethonium

    A has ganglion blocking activity
    B has a prolonged action in the presence of anticholinesterases
    C is a non-depolarising muscle relaxant
    D has a longer duration of action than d-tubocurarine
    E is given in a combined injection with thiopentone for induction of anaesthesia

---

A FALSE Succinylcholine, as suxamethonium is also known, is effectively two molecules of acetylcholine, and as such possesses, not ganglion blocking activity, but ganglion stimulating properties. This may cause peripheral vasoconstriction and lead to a rise in blood pressure.

$$CH_3\text{—}N^+\text{—}CH_2\text{—}CH_2\text{—}OC\text{—}CH_2\text{—}CH_2\text{—}CO\text{—}CH_2\text{—}CH_2\text{—}N^+\text{—}CH_3$$

suxamethonium (succinylcholine)

$$CH_3\text{—}N^+\text{—}CH_2\text{—}CH_2\text{—}OC\text{—}CH_3$$

acetylcholine

B TRUE Suxamethonium is a choline ester, and provides a suitable substrate for cholinesterase. This limits the duration of action following a therapeutic dose to about 5 minutes. In the presence of an anticholinesterase its action is dramatically prolonged.

C FALSE Like acetylcholine, suxamethonium produces depolarisation of the endplate. This causes fasciculation (random twitching) of the muscles to occur before loss of sensitivity to the endplate and paralysis ensue.

D FALSE d-tubocurarine acts for 20 to 30 minutes, whilst suxamethonium is only effective for 5 minutes (see B).

E FALSE Suxamethonium is commonly given to patients following induction of anaesthesia with thiopentone. This may be necessary to relieve the laryngospasm which sometimes occurs, but in any case it facilitates introduction of an endo-tracheal tube for the administration of a volatile anaesthetic. Under no circum-stances should suxamethonium be added to thiopentone, since the alkaline reaction of the latter inactivates the suxamethonium, and the solution becomes cloudy.

69 Suxamethonium in a small proportion of the population is particularly dangerous because

      A respiration is depressed centrally
      B hydrolysis of the drug is impaired
      C the drug is less readily excreted by the kidney
      D its action is potentiated
      E its action is prolonged

Note: The duration of action and potency of suxamethonium in the body are normally limited by the action of the pseudocholinesterase enzyme. About 1 in 4,000 of the population have an inherited enzyme defect that extends the metabolism from the usual 5 minutes to 24 hours or longer.

A FALSE The primary action of suxamethonium is to produce a depolarising blockade at the neuromuscular junction. This will include the respiratory muscles and respiration will cease. In patients with the abnormal pseudocholinesterase this may last many hours. There is no evidence, however, for any central action, and indeed with a quaternary structure one would not expect much suxamethonium to enter the brain.

B TRUE Suxamethonium is normally rapidly hydrolysed by pseudocholinesterase in the liver and plasma. The initial metabolite is succinylmonocholine which is in turn hydrolysed more slowly to succinic acid and choline. About 10 per cent of the drug is excreted unchanged, but in the presence of the abnormal enzyme this route becomes more important.

C FALSE On the contrary (see B) more drug may be excreted unchanged by this route.

D TRUE Because suxamethonium is given intravenously and cholinesterase is present in the plasma, metabolism will start immediately after injection. This limits the extent of action of suxamethonium, and in deficient individuals a much greater effect occurs. Care must also be taken following use of the intravenous induction agent propanidid which also potentiates the action of suxamethonium.

E TRUE See Note and D.

70 Which of the following statements about neuromuscular blockade is/are correct

    A tetracyclines have curare-like activity
    B pancuronium is a non-depolarising neuromuscular blocking drug
    C endrophonium is a non-depolarising neuromuscular blocking drug
    D hexamethonium is a depolarising blocker
    E direct excitability of the muscle is *unaffected* by curare blockade

---

A FALSE Aminoglycoside antibiotics like neomycin and streptomycin and some polypeptide antibiotics like polymyxin B have curare-like activity. Under rare circumstances they may potentiate the action of curare. This is not so of the tetracyclines.

B TRUE Pancuronium is a steroid molecule with a quaternary ammonium structure that produces a competitive non-depolarising neuromuscular block.

C FALSE Edrophonium has short lasting anticholinesterase activity but also stimulates directly nicotinic receptors on skeletal muscle. In small doses this can cause fasciculations, but in higher doses a depolarising block may occur.

D FALSE Hexamethonium is a ganglion blocking agent, and although structurally related to decamethonium which is a depolarising neuromuscular blocking drug, it has no neuromuscular blocking activity itself.

$$CH_3 - N^+ - (CH_2)_n - N^+ - CH_3$$

with CH_3 groups on each nitrogen.

hexamethonium n = 6
decamethonium n = 10

E TRUE Curare blocks the nicotinic receptors on which acetylcholine would normally act to induce muscle contraction. The capability of the muscle to contract following direct, i.e. electrical, stimulation would be unaffected.

71 Edrophonium

    A is a useful treatment for myasthenia gravis
    B has neuromuscular blocking activity
    C is a ganglion stimulant
    D provides a substrate for cholinesterase
    E is an anticholinesterase

A FALSE Edrophonium is an anticholinesterase drug but with a very transient action. It is therefore suitable for the diagnosis of myasthenia gravis but not its treatment. It can, however, be used to distinguish whether a myasthenic patient who is being treated with a longer acting anticholinesterase, e.g. neostigmine, is entering a 'cholinergic crisis' or a deteriorating myasthenic state. In the former edrophonium will produce a brief worsening of the condition, whilst in the latter a transient improvement will occur.

B TRUE Although normally used to diagnose myasthenia (see A) and to reverse curare blockade, because edrophonium produces direct nicotinic stimulation, as well as inhibiting cholinesterase, when used alone it will depolarise the neuromuscular junction. At low doses this may cause fasciculations, but at higher doses a depolarising block can occur.

C TRUE The stimulation of nicotinic receptors is also extended to the ganglia and this drug produces a number of resultant autonomic changes, e.g. slowing of pulse, constriction of pupil, increased peristalsis.

D FALSE Unlike neostigmine and acetylcholine, edrophonium is not metabolised by its interaction with cholinesterase. It simply complexes with the enzyme to produce inhibition.

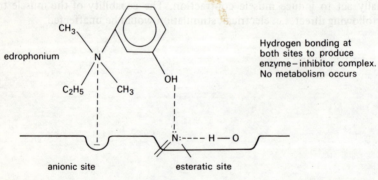

acetylcholinesterase

E TRUE See A and D.

72 The local anaesthetic lignocaine inhibits

 A conduction of nerve impulses
 B generation of nerve impulses
 C re-uptake of noradrenaline in nerve endings
 D sodium flux across nerve membranes
 E the action of sulphonamides

A TRUE The localised loss of pain and other sensations induced by local anaesthetics is due to their ability to prevent conduction of impulses along the sensory nerves which would normally convey this information to the cns.

B TRUE In addition to preventing conduction of impulses along nerves, it has been shown that local anaesthetics will inhibit generation of impulses from the free nerve endings involved in pain perception and from the receptors mediating perception of other sensations. The underlying mechanism appears to be similar (see D).

C FALSE Re-uptake of noradrenaline back into the nerves from which it has been released is the mechanism by which the transmitter action is limited in adrenergic neurones. Cocaine will block this re-uptake, thus potentiating sympathetic and central adrenergic-mediated effects. Lignocaine does not have this action.

D TRUE Initiation and passage of nerve impulses is characterised by a wave of depolarisation passing along the axon. The depolarisation is the result of efflux of potassium ions and influx of sodium ions. Local anaesthetics stabilise the membrane, perhaps by increasing the surface pressure of the lipid layer, and so hinder ionic and in particular Na^+ flux into the nerve. Nerve conduction is thus halted.

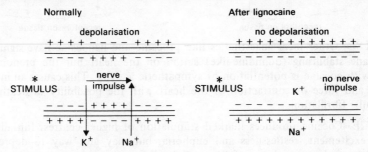

E FALSE Local anaesthetics like procaine that are derivatives of para-aminobenzoic acid (PABA) are metabolised by cholinesterase to the parent PABA, which can antagonise the cytostatic action of the sulphonamides. Lignocaine is a synthetic anilide derivative that is destroyed in the liver. The metabolites do not antagonise sulphonamide action.

73 Cocaine

    A is a useful anaesthetic for infiltration anaesthesia (i.e. by injection around nerve endings)

    B is a vasoconstrictor

    C produces a quinidine-like action on the heart

    D has a stimulant action on the cns

    E is well absorbed through mucous membranes

A FALSE The addictive potential and the systemic toxicity of cocaine (see C and D) preclude its use by injection.

B TRUE By blocking the re-uptake of noradrenaline into adrenergic nerves, cocaine prolongs and potentiates the normal sympathetic responses at both α and β-receptor sites.

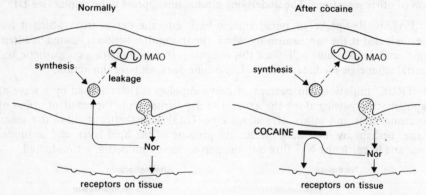

C FALSE Other local anaesthetics like procaine and lignocaine have significant membrane stabilising (quinidine-like) action on the heart but the predominant effect with cocaine is potentiation of sympathetic activity. This causes an increase in rate and force of contraction of the heart with the possibility of death from ventricular fibrillation.

D TRUE Cocaine produces marked stimulation of higher centres. Initially this causes excitement, restlessness and euphoria, but may give way to depression, medullary paralysis, respiratory failure and death.

E TRUE Cocaine is an outstandingly effective surface anaesthetic and is well absorbed through mucous membranes of the eye, buccal cavity and pharynx and is still used topically at these sites by opthalmologists and ear, nose and throat surgeons (but see A).

LOCAL ANAESTHETICS

74 Procaine

A is hydrolysed by plasma pseudocholinesterase
B reduces the efficacy of sulphonamides
C has increased efficacy when given with a vasoconstrictor
D is *not* absorbed through mucous membranes
E does *not* inhibit conduction in myelinated fibres

A TRUE Procaine provides a substrate for plasma pseudocholinesterase by which it is metabolised to para-amino-benzoic acid (PABA). Its duration of action is therefore short (see equation Q14B, page 31).

B TRUE Sulphonamides are effective by virtue of their ability to compete with PABA. This reduces bacterial synthesis of folic acid and brings about a bacteriostatic effect. The product of procaine metabolism is PABA (see A) which will compete with the sulphonamides to overcome their action. Under some circumstances this is clinically significant.

C TRUE Procaine is a vasodilator and has a rather transient effect. Adrenaline is normally added as a vasoconstrictor to prolong its action.

D TRUE Except in alkaline solution which is irritant, procaine does not readily penetrate mucous membranes.

E FALSE Local anaesthetics will block conduction in all accessible nerves whether myelinated or unmyelinated. Under normal use a differential action is seen simply because the finer unmyelinated pain fibres are penetrated most readily. Touch, temperature, pressure and proprioceptive senses are systematically affected in order of increasing fibre diameter, and at higher concentrations even somatic nerves are blocked.

75 When producing local anaesthesia by infiltration

    A amethocaine is a suitable alternative in patients who are allergic to lignocaine

    B the duration of anaesthesia may be prolonged by addition of adrenaline

    C the rate of absorption of the drug into the bloodstream can be increased by addition of felypressin

    D adrenaline-containing anaesthetic preparations should be avoided in patients receiving tricyclic antidepressants

    E inadvertent injection of lignocaine into the general circulation will increase myocardial excitability and may cause arrhythmias

---

A FALSE Hypersensitivity to lignocaine is very rare, but amethocaine should not be used as an alternative; it is too toxic for injection and even when used for surface anaesthesia can cause sensitisation.

B TRUE The duration of anaesthesia produced by local anaesthetics is dependent primarily on the rate at which they are removed from the site of injection. Vasoconstrictor agents like adrenaline, by reducing the local circulation, prevent the anaesthetic from diffusing away and prolong their effect.

C FALSE Felypressin is a synthetic analogue of the pituitary peptide hormone vasopressin. It has vasoconstrictor properties and when added to a local anaesthetic delays absorption into the bloodstream.

D TRUE Adrenaline when injected into the circulation is removed primarily by uptake into the tissues (some is broken down by the enzyme catechol-O-methyl transferase (COMT)). Tricyclic antidepressants by blocking the re-uptake process (Uptake 1) might therefore be expected to potentiate the actions of adrenaline. This has been demonstrated experimentally in human volunteers, but whether it would occur if a local anaesthetic containing adrenaline was inadvertently injected into a vein is uncertain. The advice is generally not to take the risk.

E FALSE Lignocaine has a quinidine-like action on the heart to reduce excitability and is given intravenously to treat cardiac arrhythmias. Amongst the local anaesthetics only cocaine causes increased excitability of the heart and since this may lead to ventricular fibrillation, it should never be injected into a patient.

Local Anaesthetics: related questions 99, 100

76 An increase in heart rate characteristically follows clinical use of which of the following drugs

    A bethanecol
    B digitoxin
    C glyceryl trinitrate
    D isoprenaline
    E sotalol

A FALSE A parasympathomimetic, resistant to the action of cholinesterase, bethanecol produces primarily muscarinic action including bradycardia.

B FALSE Apart from its positive inotropic effect on cardiac muscle, digitoxin will normally slow the heart rate, especially if the initial rate is high (as in failure). It is thought to do this in a number of ways. First, it stimulates the brain stem to increase vagal activity, secondly, it effects a sensitisation of pacemaker cells and Purkinje fibres to the action of acetylcholine, and thirdly, it lowers the threshold of baroreceptors so that reflex bradycardia will occur at a lower systemic blood pressure.

C TRUE Glyceryl trinitrate by dilating peripheral blood vessels lowers the blood pressure and this induces a reflex tachycardia.

D TRUE Isoprenaline can be used with the deliberate intention of increasing heart rate, e.g. to improve cardiac output in complete heart block: on the other hand, tachycardia may simply occur as an unwanted side effect, e.g. during use as a bronchodilator.

E FALSE Sotalol is a β-adrenoceptor antagonist which will prevent the action of sympathetic amines on the heart, therefore in the presence of sympathetic stimulation lowering the heart rate.

77 Relaxation of arterioles in the skin and splanchnic areas of the body

    A is a useful method for relieving angina of effort
    B may be induced with salbutamol
    C may be induced with hydralazine
    D occurs when a tobacco is smoked by a regular smoker
    E follows the injection of felypressin

A TRUE The pain of angina of effort is due to a transient oxygen deficiency in the myocardium. It may be relieved by reducing the work load on the heart, and this can be achieved by reducing the peripheral resistance, i.e. relaxation of peripheral arterioles and venules. This is the mechanism of action of the nitrates and nitrites.

B FALSE Salbutamol is a selective β_2-stimulant and may cause dilatation of blood vessels in skeletal muscle. However, primarily α-adrenoceptors are present in the skin and splanchnic area and stimulation of these would cause vasoconstriction.

C TRUE Hydralazine produces a profound fall in arteriolar tone in the skin and splanchnic area. It is used in severe hypertension and has the advantage that the renal blood flow is not impaired. It appears to act directly on the arterioles.

D FALSE The nicotine absorbed from tobacco smoke by stimulating autonomic ganglia and by releasing adrenaline from the adrenal medulla produces vasoconstriction of peripheral arterioles. Smoking aggravates conditions where peripheral circulation is impaired.

E FALSE Felypressin is a synthetic analogue of the pituitary peptide hormone vasopressin. It produces vasoconstriction by a direct action of arteriolar smooth muscle and is added to the local anaesthetic prilocaine to delay its absorption. It has the advantage of producing no direct action on the heart and of not being potentiated by tricyclic or monoamine oxidase antidepressant therapy.

78 Typically, following administration to man one would expect
- A glyceryl trinitrate to produce a dramatic flush within 30 seconds
- B cigarette smoking to produce a decrease in pulse rate and blood pressure
- C phenylephrine to constrict the pupil
- D isoprenaline to increase dramatically the FEV_1 in non-asthmatic subjects
- E metoprolol to inhibit exercise-induced tachycardia

A FALSE Glyceryl trinitrate is normally administered sublingually to escape destruction in the liver. It produces peripheral dilation which develops over several minutes and which lasts for half an hour or more. An immediate flush of the type described is produced by the volatile inhalation agent amyl nitrite.

B FALSE The average cigarette when smoked may yield 6 to 8 mg of nicotine, but the amount that enters the body will depend on how it is smoked. Up to 90 per cent of nicotine inhaled into the lungs may be absorbed whilst only 25 to 50 per cent will be absorbed from smoke held in the mouth. The nicotine will stimulate ganglia the primary effects of which are vasoconstriction and release of adrenaline and noradrenaline from the adrenal medulla. This usually causes a tachycardia and a rise in both systolic and diastolic blood pressure, although the extent will depend on the amount of nicotine consumed.

C FALSE Phenylephrine is a direct α-adrenoceptor stimulant, and if applied to the eye would induce pupillary dilatation, by causing contraction of the dilator pupillae.

D FALSE The forced expiratory volume in one second (FEV_1) is the volume of air displaced from the lungs when expiration is carried out as rapidly as possible following a maximal inspiration. In a normal healthy subject at least 75 per cent of the total volume of air expired in this manner (the so-called forced vital capacity), is removed in the first second, indicating good compliance of the airways. In asthmatics it may be reduced to as little as 40 per cent, and although in these patients isoprenaline will increase this towards normal levels, it has no significant effect on the airways resistance of normal subjects.

E TRUE The heart rate increase induced by exercise is due to reflex release of noradrenaline from sympathetic nerves and of adrenaline from the adrenal medulla. Metoprolol is a selective β_1-blocker and will therefore prevent the chronotropic action of these amines on the heart.

79 The benefits of dopamine therapy in cardiogenic shock include
- A a rise in diastolic blood pressure
- B arteriolar constriction
- C slowing of the heart
- D increased force of cardiac contraction
- E vasodilatation in the kidneys

A FALSE Although between 50 to 250 times less potent, like adrenaline, dopamine stimulates directly both α and β-receptors. It also stimulates dopaminergic receptors in the kidney and mesenteric areas (see E). The overall effect is one of vasodilatation, and when given at a rate of up to about 3 μg/kg/min dopamine ensures adequate tissue perfusion, especially of the kidneys. Fluids should be infused to counteract the fall in blood pressure. At higher infusion rates (3 to 10 μg/kg/min), an inotropic action on the heart is produced (see D), but in amounts greater than this powerful vasoconstriction may occur, with the possibility of gangrene.

B FALSE See A.

C FALSE Dopamine stimulates β-receptors, but compared with other catecholamines the increase in heart rate for a given increase in force of cardiac contraction is much less. This means that dangerous tachycardias and arrhythmias are less likely.

D TRUE Dopamine has a direct positive inotropic action on the heart so that cardiac output is increased. The advantage of dopamine is that it produces less tachycardia than other catecholamines (see C). As a result of its action systolic blood pressure will rise.

E TRUE By stimulating dopaminergic receptors in the kidney, dopamine induces a powerful vasodilatation. This effect is not blocked by α or β-antagonists, and leads to improvement of renal function and increased urine output. Similar dopaminergic receptors are thought to be present in the coronary and intracerebral vasculature.

80 In the clinical management of migraine

    A methysergide is used as a prophylactic
    B ergotamine powder may be administered by aerosol inhaler
    C aspirin is of value in mild attacks
    D clonidine is effective
    E the contraceptive pill increases the frequency of attacks

A TRUE 5-hydroxytryptamine (5-HT) has been implicated in the initial vaso-constrictor phase that precedes the vasodilatation and increased pulse pressure associated with migrainous headaches. The 5-HT antagonist methysergide has thus been used prophylactically in an attempt to forestall these events.

B TRUE When administered orally ergotamine absorption is unreliable, and more consistent results can be achieved by inhalation of the ergotamine powder from an aerosol inhaler.

C TRUE The pain of *mild* attacks can be controlled in many patients by using aspirin or paracetamol, although if nausea is troublesome an antiemetic may be needed in addition.

D TRUE Clonidine, like methysergide, is used as a prophylactic. It probably acts by reducing the responsiveness of blood vessels to vasoactive substances and thus interrupts the sequence of events leading to migraine. It is used at lower doses than employed for control of hypertension.

E TRUE Use of the contraceptive pill is associated with about a two-fold increase in the incidence of migraine.

Cardiovascular System — General: related questions 30, 38, 39, 40, 50, 52, 143, 144, 145, 146

81 Which of the following drugs lower blood pressure *primarily by a direct action* **on sympathetic postganglionic nerves to reduce noradrenaline output**

    A propranolol
    B diazoxide
    C reserpine
    D guanethidine
    E clonidine

A FALSE Propranolol is a β-blocker used mainly in the treatment of hypertension and angina pectoris. It prevents sympathetic stimulation of the heart by antagonising the action of released transmitter on β-adrenoceptors. It also has a central action to reduce overall sympathetic tone, but it has no direct action on sympathetic nerves.

B FALSE A derivative of the thiazide diuretics, diazoxide is a potent vasodilator when given intravenously. It acts directly on vascular smooth muscle to produce hypotension lasting about 12 hours. It is used to treat hypertensive crises.

C TRUE Reserpine brings about a rapid depletion of neuronal stores, so that the output of noradrenaline following nerve stimulation is reduced. The depleted amine is deaminated by monoamine oxidase (MAO) before release from the nerve so that it does not produce a pharmacological effect. The main action seems to be to block the uptake of noradrenaline into vesicles. Since the vesicles are leaky, noradrenaline

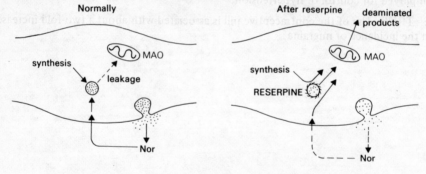

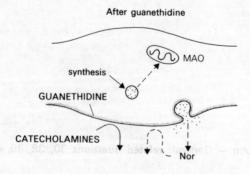

is lost into the cytosol and any taken back into the nerve following nerve exocytosis will also remain in the cytosol. This noradrenaline will be metabolised by mitochondrial MAO. Reserpine has important central actions but they are not thought to contribute to the reduction of sympathetic nerve effects.

D TRUE Guanethidine is the classic adrenergic neurone blocking agent that prevents release of noradrenaline from sympathetic nerves. After a period of treatment or following high doses it also brings about depletion of neuronal stores. The precise mechanism is unclear, but guanethidine has an action on the neuronal membrane that prevents normal transmitter release probably by competing with Ca^{++} in the excitation-secretion coupling. It also prevents uptake of amines into the nerve, an action that causes supersensitivity to administered catecholamines.

E FALSE Clonidine has a small guanethidine-like effect, but most of its action appears to be mediated centrally to reduce both constrictor tone in blood vessels and sympathetic drive to the heart. The primary site of action is the medullary vasomotor centre where stimulation of α-receptors occurs.

82 In the treatment of essential hypertension

    A chlorothiazide is useful because it depresses the cardiovascular centre
    B α-methyl dopa blocks α-receptors
    C α-blockers like phentolamine are useful
    D labetalol blocks α-receptors
    E ganglionic blockers are the drugs of choice

A FALSE Chlorothiazide is diuretic and hypotensive. Its primary site of action is on the kidney to inhibit Na^+ reabsorption and although this causes an initial reduction of blood volume it cannot effectively explain the hypotension, since plasma volume returns to pretreatment levels whilst hypotension continues. This appears to be due to dilatation of peripheral blood vessels by a direct action of the drug on vascular smooth muscle. The exact mechanism is not clear, but it has been suggested that a decreased sodium content in the arterial walls alters its reactivity to endogenous constrictor substances. There is no evidence for a centrally mediated action.

B FALSE α-methyl dopa is converted by dopa decarboxylase in adrenergic neurones to α-methyl dopamine, which in turn is converted by dopamine-β-hydroxylase to α-methyl noradrenaline. This, it is thought, stimulates α-receptors in the cardiovascular centre to effect a reduction in sympathetic tone. α-methyl noradrenaline on the periphery is a vasoconstrictor and neither this nor α-methyl dopa is thought to block α-receptors.

C FALSE Although α-receptor stimulation causes vasoconstriction with a rise in peripheral resistance, and blockade of the sympathetic system is an important method in the control of hypertension, results with pure α-blocking agents have been disappointing. An important factor is that β-receptors are unaffected, so that reflex tachycardia occurs, which added to toxicity of the individual agents has made them generally unacceptable for widespread use. Furthermore, drugs like phentolamine block both pre and postjunctional α-receptors which may lead to increased output of noradrenaline from the nerves and in turn reduce the effectiveness of the blockade. The drug prazosin, which only blocks postjunctional receptors produces a useful hypotensive action.

D TRUE The '-olol' and '-alol' endings describe drugs which have β-blocking activity, but labetalol is unique in that it blocks in addition α-adrenoceptors. This means that the reduction in peripheral resistance that it produces is not followed by a reflex tachycardia (see C), and the drug can be used to treat hypertension.

E FALSE Ganglion blocking agents by blocking transmission throughout the autonomic nervous system, produce not only a fall in blood pressure but also a host of other unwanted effects. These include dry mouth, constipation, inability to accommodate for near vision, urinary retention, impotence etc. They are only rarely used.

83 Ganglionic blocking agents (GBAs) are not prescribed in the long term management of essential hypertension because they

    A produce only a trivial lowering of blood pressure
    B cause diarrhoea
    C bring about accommodation for near vision
    D cause postural hypotension
    E cause impotence

A FALSE At full therapeutic doses ganglion blocking drugs produce excellent lowering of blood pressure, but the very mechanism by which such profound effects are obtained, i.e. blockade of all ganglia in the autonomic nervous system, causes a number of unwanted side effects (see B, C, D and E).

B FALSE Stimulation of sympathetic nerves to the gastrointestinal tract inhibits movement and lowers tone; stimulation of parasympathetic nerves causes contraction and raises tone. However, the parasympathetic influences normally predominate and ganglionic blockade leads to gut stasis and constipation.

C FALSE Stimulation of parasympathetic nerves supplying the ciliary muscle causes them to contract. This pulls in the ciliary body so relaxing the suspensory ligament in such a way that the lens bulges and the eye accommodates for near vision. GBAs by interfering with transmission will prevent this process.

D TRUE In a sitting or lying position blood tends to pool in the lower part of the body. In order to maintain the blood pressure on standing (as detected by the carotid sinus) reflex vasoconstriction occurs in arterioles, venules and veins and a slight rise in heart rate occurs. GBAs block the efferent arc of this reflex and so cause postural hypotension.

E TRUE Sexual performance in the male is totally dependent on a normally functioning autonomic nerve supply to the sex organs. Penile erection is under parasympathetic control and ejaculation under sympathetic control, and any interference with the nerve supply is likely to cause impotence. GBAs prevent both erection and ejaculation, whereas antihypertensive agents showing specificity for the adrenergic neurone may only prevent ejaculation.

84 Diastolic blood pressure falls following administration of α-methyl dopa because

    A the sympathetic system is depressed centrally
    B sympathetic ganglia are blocked
    C it reduces peripheral resistance
    D a false transmitter is synthesised
    E α-methyl dopa is an adrenergic blocker

A TRUE α-methyl dopa is converted to α-methyl noradrenaline (see D) which by stimulating α-adrenoceptors in the vasomotor centre (vmc) is thought to effect the reduction in sympathetic tone which occurs. The action of α-methyl noradrenaline on the vmc is blocked by the α-blocker phentolamine.

B FALSE Transmission at ganglia is cholinergic (nicotinic) and there is no evidence that α-methyl dopa produces a significant action at this site.

C TRUE Most drugs used in the treatment of hypertension that lower diastolic blood pressure do so by effecting a reduction in vasomotor tone in resistance vessels throughout the body. α-methyl dopa is no exception.

D TRUE α-methyl dopa is converted to the false transmitter α-methyl noradrenaline. Its primary action is central (see A) but a peripheral action cannot be ruled out.

$$\alpha\text{-methyl-dopa} \xrightarrow[\text{decarboxylase}]{\text{dopa}} \alpha\text{-methyl dopamine} \xrightarrow[\beta\text{-hydroxylase}]{\text{dopamine}} \alpha\text{-methyl noradrenaline}$$

E FALSE α-methyl dopa is effective because it is converted to α-methyl noradrenaline (see A and D), not because it possesses important adrenergic blocking activity.

85 Guanethidine lowers systemic blood pressure by an action

    A on autonomic ganglia
    B to block β-receptors
    C to prevent release of adrenergic neurotransmitter
    D to deplete the adrenergic nerve ending of transmitter
    E directly on the smooth muscle of the arterioles

A FALSE Transmission at autonomic ganglia of both the sympathetic and para-sympathetic systems is cholinergic, and although adrenergic neurone blocking agents like guanethidine have local anaesthetic activity, they do not interfere with transmission at this site. Because of their greater specificity of action the range of side effects they produce are less than those seen with ganglion blocking agents.

B FALSE Quite the contrary, by preventing the uptake of sympathomimetic amines into the neurone, guanethidine potentiates both the α and β actions of injected amines.

C TRUE When guanethidine is administered, there is commonly a transient sympathomimetic action due to noradrenaline release from the nerve ending, but this is followed by a blockade in which depolarisation of the nerve no longer causes noradrenaline release. This is apparently due to the drug competing with Ca^{++} ions in excitation-secretion coupling. Guanethidine also blocks the uptake of amines into the nerve (see B and diagram Q81C, page 100).

D TRUE Following prolonged administration or high doses of guanethidine, neuronal stores of amine become depleted. Some of the amine is deaminated before release but some escapes unchanged and may, by producing sympathomimetic effects, limit the usefulness of the drug. Depletion of stores persists for many days after treatment has stopped.

E FALSE There is no evidence that guanethidine produces a significant direct action on the smooth muscle of the arterioles.

86 The antihypertensive drug, guanethidine

A is a sympathetic α-blocker
B does not cause postural hypotension
C has important actions on the cns
D may have its action abolished by concurrent administration of phenyl-butazone
E may have its action abolished by concurrent administration of desipramine

---

A FALSE   Guanethidine does not possess α-blocking activity, a fact that is readily demonstrated by the supersensitivity that occurs when sympathomimetic drugs are given in its presence. Guanethidine is taken up into nerves by the Uptake 1 process: this effectively blocks the system so that agents like noradrenaline produce a greater than normal action.

B FALSE   As with all drugs interfering with the sympathetic vasoconstrictor processes which would normally operate when moving from a sitting or lying position to standing, guanethidine produces postural hypotension.

C FALSE   Unlike most other drugs used in the treatment of hypertension guanethidine does not cross the blood/brain barrier.

D TRUE   By an action on the renal tubules phenylbutazone causes Na^+ and water retention with a consequent increase in plasma volume. Control of hypertension by guanethidine will as a result be lost.

E TRUE   Desipramine is a tricyclic antidepressant drug that inhibits re-uptake of noradrenaline into adrenergic neurones, so potentiating the action of noradrenaline. For guanethidine to be effective as an antihypertensive agent, it too must be taken up into the sympathetic neurones (see A). Desipramine and a variety of other drugs, by blocking the uptake of guanethidine, will antagonise its hypertensive action.

87 Several mechanisms are involved in the hypotensive action of clonidine. They include

    A decreased sympathetic outflow from the cns
    B ganglionic blockade
    C adrenergic blockade
    D reduced reactivity of arteriolar smooth muscle
    E sodium and water depletion

A TRUE The primary site of action of clonidine is thought to be the vasomotor centre in the cns where by stimulating α-receptors it causes a reduction in sympathetic tone and thus hypotension and bradycardia.

B FALSE Although several mechanisms are involved in the hypotensive effect of clonidine, ganglionic blockade is not thought to occur. The dry mouth, drowsiness and constipation are centrally mediated effects.

C FALSE Clonidine is chemically related to the α-blocker tolazoline, but stimulation of α-adrenoceptors rather than blockade is the predominant but transient peripheral effect. Vasoconstriction following intravenous injection, occurs briefly in animal experiments because of this action (see also D).

D TRUE There is some evidence that, in addition to its central action, clonidine reduces the sensitivity of peripheral arteriolar walls to the vasoconstrictor actions of angiotensin and circulating catecholamines.

E FALSE Clonidine does not have a diuretic action, and is most effective clinically when combined with a diuretic.

88 Which of the following is/are essential to the hypotensive action of thiazides

    A depletion of body potassium
    B a direct effect on the arteriolar wall
    C inhibition of the vasomotor centre in the cns
    D reduction in renin release
    E reduction in cardiac output

A FALSE Some of the thiazides, like chlorothiazide, have important diuretic properties, whilst others, like diazoxide, which are not diuretic may actually decrease sodium and water excretion. The diuretic ones do produce hypokalaemia but this is not thought to be of importance in lowering the blood pressure.

B TRUE Both chlorothiazide and diazoxide have a direct action on arterioles to produce relaxation and to reduce their responsiveness to vasoconstrictor agents. There is no postural element to the hypotension which suggests that they do not affect post-capillary capacitance vessels.

C FALSE The available evidence suggests that the hypotensive action of the thiazides is peripheral (see B) and not on the cns.

D FALSE The reduced blood volume (see E) and blood pressure induced by thiazides may in some individuals be sufficient to impair perfusion in the afferent glomerular arterioles in the kidney and thus lead to release of renin from the juxta-glomerular apparatus. By effecting production of angiotensin and in turn the release of aldosterone from the adrenal gland the blood volume may increase and the blood pressure rise, thus negating the action of the diuretic.

E FALSE Because of the diuretic action of chlorothiazide there is an initial fall in circulating blood volume with a resulting fall in cardiac output. However, this does not appear to be an essential part of the mechanism of action of thiazides. First, diazoxide which is not diuretic is effective, and secondly, the blood volume after prolonged treatment with chlorothiazide may return to normal without loss of hypotensive effect. The cardiac output may well then increase.

89 In the management of essential hypertension

    A β-blockers are *in*appropriate therapy
    B the diuretic chlorothiazide is effective in mild disease
    C reserpine is effective because it inhibits monoamine oxidase (MAO)
    D hydralazine is an adrenergic neurone blocker
    E α-methyl dopa acts through its ability to inhibit dopamine β-hydroxy-lase

---

A FALSE β-blockers like propranolol are widely used in the management of hypertension, although their mechanism of action is far from clear. In the short term by reducing sympathetic drive to the heart they decrease cardiac output and thus systolic blood pressure; but a central action on the cardiovascular centre to effect an overall reduction in sympathetic tone (especially to peripheral blood vessels) is more important. Other possible contributory actions include a reduction in renin release from the kidney and long term adaptation of the peripheral resistance to a reduced cardiac output.

B TRUE Chlorothiazide is effective in mild hypertension but its mechanism of action is unclear. The reduction in blood volume it produces initially as a result of its diuretic action does not account for all of its effect, because the hypotensive action continues after the blood volume has returned to its pretreatment value. Alteration of the Na^+ content of peripheral blood vessels, and hence their sensitivity to constrictor influences seems a more likely explanation.

C FALSE Reserpine is an effective but not widely used hypotensive agent, that acts by virtue of its ability to deplete neuronal stores of noradrenaline. It acts on the vesicles and the amine which escapes is metabolised by mitochondrial MAO, so that sympathomimetic effects do not occur.

D FALSE Hydralazine has a direct action on peripheral arterioles to cause dilatation and to reduce vascular reactivity. It has no central action, has little effect on the venous system and produces little postural hypotension. A slight reflex tachycardia may occur.

E FALSE α-methyl dopa is converted by the action of the enzyme dopa decarboxylase to α-methyl noradrenaline, which acts centrally on α-adrenoceptors to reduce sympathetic tone. At the periphery the conversion of α-methyl dopa to α-methyl noradrenaline reduces the synthesis of noradrenaline, partly by providing an alternative substrate and partly by inhibiting the dopa decarboxylase. There is no evidence for an important action on dopamine β-hydroxylase.

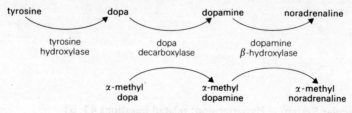

90 The toxicity of hydralazine includes

A impotence
B systemic lupus erythematosus
C tachycardia
D constipation
E difficulty in accommodating for near vision

Note: Hydralazine acts directly on the arterioles to cause vasodilatation and to reduce the vascular response to constrictor agents By not interfering with autonomic nerve function elsewhere in the body, many of the complicating features of antihypertensive therapy are not seen.

A FALSE Sexual performance in the male requires a functionally intact autonomic nervous system; the parasympathetic to produce erection and the sympathetic to bring about ejaculation. Since hydralazine affects neither, impotence does not occur.

B TRUE Following prolonged use of large doses of hydralazine a condition resembling either early rheumatoid arthritis or systemic lupus erythematosus (SLE) may occur. An immunological basis for its incidence has been suggested, but it is more likely to occur in subjects who are slow acetylators. The condition is usually reversible on stopping treatment, but severe SLE may require prolonged treatment with corticosteroids.

C TRUE Marked tachycardia and palpitations are common features of treatment and are thought to be due to the reflex which follows the fall in blood pressure. Small doses injected into the cerebral ventricles in animals has a similar effect which might suggest a central action as well. Either way, the effect can be prevented by β-blockers.

D FALSE Constipation is a feature of autonomic and especially parasympathetic blockade, and commonly follows treatment with ganglion blocking agents. It is not seen with hydralazine.

E FALSE Accommodation for near vision is under parasympathetic control and is therefore unaffected by treatment with hydralazine.

Cardiovascular System — Hypertension: related questions 41, 51

91 Which of the following drugs is useful in the treatment of angina pectoris

    A quinidine
    B quinine
    C propranolol
    D salbutamol
    E digoxin

A FALSE Quinidine is an antidysrhythmic drug that decreases myocardial excitability, prolongs the refractory period, and decreases conduction velocity. It also has weak vasodilator actions, and although it might succeed in producing some of the properties required of an antianginal drug, it is a toxic drug and its use is reserved for the prevention and abolition of cardiac dysrythmias.

B FALSE Quinine is a seldom used antimalarial drug with some small quinidine like actions (see A).

C TRUE The β-blocker propranolol, by virtue of its ability to block both sympathetic drive to, and the effects of circulating adrenaline on, the heart will reduce heart rate and thus the oxygen demands of the myocardium. This in turn will relieve the associated pain. Propranolol is widely used in the treatment of angina.

D FALSE Salbutamol is a selective β_2 stimulant used to induce bronchodilatation in asthmatics. It has minimal cardiac effects at normal therapeutic doses, but at higher doses it stimulates the heart. This is the opposite effect to that required of an antianginal drug.

E FALSE Digoxin is a cardiac glycoside that slows heart rate and increases the force of cardiac contraction. It is used to treat heart failure and certain abnormal rhythms.

92 Glyceryl trinitrate is effective in the treatment of angina because it

    A dilates the coronary arteries
    B dilates peripheral arterioles
    C slows the heart
    D stimulates β-receptors
    E causes reduction of oxygen consumption by the myocardium

---

A FALSE In angina the coronary arteries are atherosclerotic and therefore limit the blood through the coronary tree, irrespective of the state of dilatation of the coronary arterioles. The atherosclerotic coronary arteries cannot dilate.

B TRUE Glyceryl trinitrate induces relaxation of smooth muscle in a number of tissues. In angina the most important effect is dilatation of peripheral blood vessels (not only arterioles but also veins and venules) which lowers the peripheral resistance and allows pooling of blood in capacitance vessels. The effect is two-fold; blood pressure drops, and venous return falls, so that both pre-load and after-load on the heart are reduced. This reduces the work done by the cardiac muscle.

C FALSE Heart rate reflexly increases due to the fall in blood pressure.

D FALSE Glyceryl trinitrate has no direct action on β-receptors. In any case stimulation of β-receptors in the heart would make angina worse. Its actual cellular mechanism is uncertain, but it may involve interaction with cytochrome oxidase and a change in oxygen transfer into the cell.

E TRUE Because of the reduction of work load on the heart (see B) oxygen consumption of the myocardium falls.

93 In the treatment of angina of effort

    A glyceryl trinitrate is administered sublingually
    B propranolol is given by aerosol inhaler
    C amyl nitrite produces dilatation of venules at the periphery
    D dipyridamole acts by decreasing myocardial work
    E amyl nitrite is effective without metabolic conversion

A TRUE Following sublingual administration organic nitrates are rapidly absorbed from the buccal mucosa to give an intense and predictable effect. Rapid absorption from the gastrointestinal mucosa also follows oral administration, but 'first pass' inactivation by the liver ensures that little reaches the systemic circulation in active form. The normal route of administration is thus sublingual.

B FALSE Propranolol is used prophylactically in the treatment of angina to prevent the cardiac response to anxiety, exercise and emotion. It is readily absorbed following oral administration, and little would be achieved by use of an aerosol, a route normally reserved for local effects in the lungs.

C TRUE Amyl nitrite as with other nitrites and nitrates (see D) produces relaxation of smooth muscle throughout the body including that in the venular walls. The usefulness of these compounds is in part due to this action.

D FALSE Dipyridamole decreases coronary vascular resistance and increases coronary blood flow and coronary sinus oxygenation. The present evidence suggests that it does this by potentiating the coronary vasodilator effect of normal metabolic products such as purine nucleotides. Dipyridamole is an interesting drug because it also inhibits platelet aggregation, probably by amplifying the action of low concentrations of prostacyclin. The clinical significance of this has yet to be established.

E TRUE Amyl nitrite is effective on entering the circulation. Metabolic conversion is not required.

94 Digitalis

    A is negatively inotropic
    B inhibits central vagal connections
    C has a low therapeutic index
    D enhances excitability of the ventricular muscle
    E has an atropine-like action on cholinergic receptors in the heart

---

A FALSE Digitalis inhibits the Na^+-K^+ membrane ATPase so that intracellular Na^+ levels increase and K^+ levels fall. This has the effect of making more Ca^{++} available for the contractile mechanisms and a *positive* inotropic effect is produced.

B FALSE On the contrary, digitalis increases vagal firing by a direct action on the medullary vagal centre (see also E).

C TRUE Digitalis has a very low therapeutic ratio and toxicity is common in most patients at some stage during therapy. This may take the form of gastro-intestinal upset, visual disturbances or effects on the heart such as arrhythmia or heart block.

D TRUE As a result of the changes in intracellular Na^+ and K^+ levels (see A) the membrane potential is reduced. The effect is to increase myocardial excitability.

E FALSE Digitalis sensitises the pacemaker cells and Pürkinje fibres to the effects of acetylcholine. This, combined with an action on the medulla to increase vagal firing (see B), and a lowering of the baroreceptor threshold so that vagal slowing is triggered more easily, mean that digitalis slows the heart and reduces conduction in the bundle of His. As might be expected the action is blocked by atropine.

95 Digitalis is beneficial in the treatment of cardiac failure because it

    A increases heart rate and therefore cardiac output
    B increases conduction in the bundle of His
    C increases the force of contraction
    D reduces excitability of the myocardium
    E dilates the coronary arteries

Note: In cardiac failure the heart is incapable of maintaining an adequate cardiac output to cope with the metabolic needs of the body. If failure becomes chronic, hypertrophy of the myocardium will occur, but contractility is eventually impaired and as the heart becomes distended with blood it gets less and less able to deal with the venous return. The venous pressure rises but no longer provokes increased myocardial contractility (Starling's Law is not obeyed) and oedema occurs. The heart rate rises reflexly as a result of sympathetic drive in an attempt to improve cardiac output.

A FALSE Cardiac output does increase, but digitalis slows cardiac rate, and although this is not of value per se it allows more complete diastolic filling of the ventricles and a longer duration of recovery of the myocardium between contractions. These actions combined with increased contractility of the heart cause a dramatic improvement in cardiac output.

B FALSE Conduction through the bundle of His is reduced. This is part of the reason why cardiac rate is reduced (see A).

C TRUE The positive inotropic action of digitalis increases both the force and velocity of myocardial contraction, so that ejection of blood from the ventricles occurs both more quickly and more completely, i.e. the Starling curve returns towards normal. Cardiac output rises and diastolic filling pressure falls, effects which help to improve peripheral perfusion and to reduce oedema.

D FALSE At low doses the excitability of the myocardium is slightly *increased* due to the decreased resting potential associated with the altered ionic distribution that follows inhibition of the membrane ATPase. At increasing doses excitability is *reduced* affecting first the atria but progressing down to the ventricles. However, this may be regarded as a toxic manifestation of digitalis therapy.

E FALSE Coronary blood flow both in normal and failing hearts, is unaffected by digitalis therapy. An increase in coronary blood flow following treatment with digitalis might in any case be superfluous because oxygen demand of the myocardium falls as the cardiac cells become more efficient, i.e. as heart size is reduced and fibre tension falls.

96 Digoxin can produce

A bradycardia
B tachycardia
C heart block
D ventricular fibrillation
E atrial fibrillation

A TRUE Digoxin can produce an indirect vagal-induced bradycardia. It is seen mainly at high heart rates. It is due to a combination of three effects. First, digitalis sensitises pacemaker and Pürkinje cells to the effects of acetylcholine; secondly, there is a reduction in the baroreceptor threshold so that vagal slowing of the heart is triggered more easily; and thirdly, digitalis increases vagal firing by a direct action on the medullary centre. All three actions are blocked by atropine. The reduction in conduction through the bundle of His (see C) also contributes to the bradycardia.

B TRUE Digitalis increases the rate of spontaneous diastolic depolarisation of pacemaker cells during phase 4 of the action potential. This leads to increased automaticity especially in the ventricles. Initially, this may lead to premature systoles but at high doses tachycardia may occur. The outcome may be ventricular fibrillation (see D).

C TRUE Conduction in the bundle of His is reduced partly as a result of increased sensitivity of Pürkinje fibres to acetylcholine, and partly as a result of a change in ionic movement in the myocardial cells to reduce both the membrane potential and the rate of rise and amplitude of the action potential. If conduction is reduced sufficiently then some impulses from the sinoatrial node will arrive at the atrioventricular node and Pürkinje fibres during the refractory period of the tissue and will not be conducted to the ventricles, i.e. heart block exists.

D TRUE With increasing dosage of digitalis, heart block and complete atrioventricular dissociation may occur. Increasing automaticity of ectopic pacemaker cells in the ventricles may then lead to ventricular fibrillation.

E TRUE If digitalis is administered to man or animals in whom there is atrial flutter, then atrial fibrillation may be induced. The action is in part due to a reduction in atrial refractory period, but does not occur in the presence of atropine (after which digitalis prolongs the refractory period). Conversion of atrial flutter to fibrillation is generally considered to be useful since it facilitates control of the ventricular rate.

97 The actions of digoxin are

    A due to inhibition of ATPase
    B due to blocking of Na^+ inflow
    C diminished by low plasma K^+
    D diminished by low plasma Ca^{++}
    E due to increased excitability of the myocardium

A TRUE The positive inotropic action of digoxin is indirectly the result of in-hibition of the Na^+-K^+ membrane ATPase (the enzyme normally responsible for the expulsion of Na^+ from the cell). Accumulation of Na^+ in the cell and intra-cellular depletion of K^+ occur which facilitates the transfer of Ca^{++} into the cell and Ca^{++} release from the sarcoplasmic reticulum. The Ca^{++} by binding to tro-ponin allows actin-myosin contraction coupling to occur.

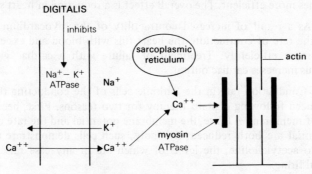

B FALSE Na^+ expulsion is blocked (see A).

C FALSE Low plasma K^+ (hypokalaemia) will enhance the efflux of K^+, reduce the transmembrane potential, enhance glycoside binding and potentiate both the pharmacological and toxic actions of digitalis.

D TRUE Low plasma Ca^{++} levels reduce the availability of Ca^{++} for the contrac-tion coupling system and digoxin action is reduced (see A).

E TRUE The altered distribution of ions (see A) that occurs with small doses of digoxin lowers the transmembrane potential and increases the excitability to electrical stimulation. This may evoke extrasystoles.

98 Following the treatment of congestive heart failure with digitoxin there is typically an increase in

    A heart size
    B cardiac output
    C conduction rate in the Pürkinje fibres
    D urine production
    E body weight

A FALSE In congestive heart failure, partly due to compensatory hypertrophy of the myocardium and partly because the heart is distended with blood, the heart is larger than normal. By increasing the force and velocity of cardiac contraction digitoxin causes ejection of blood from the ventricles to occur more quickly and more completely so that the Starling curve moves back towards normal, i.e. the heart becomes more efficient. The overall effect is a reduction in heart size.

B TRUE As a result of increased contractility of the myocardium (see A) and slowing of the rate of contraction, the heart fills with blood and expels it into the circulation more efficiently. Treatment of failure with a cardiac glycoside like digitoxin thus increases cardiac output.

C FALSE Conduction rate in the Pürkinje cells of the conducting tissues of the heart is reduced following digitalis therapy for two reasons. First, because there is inhibition of membrane ATPase, the membrane potential and the rate of rise of the action potential are both reduced. Secondly, such cells demonstrate an increased sensitivity to acetylcholine, the levels of which are in any case raised due to increased vagal firing.

D TRUE In failure, the heart no longer responds to an increase in venous pressure by increased contractility, which together with poor cardiac output leads to venous congestion and oedema. This is the classical picture of dropsy for which William Withering originally prescribed digitalis, and in which he saw such a dramatic improvement. Digitalis by improving cardiac efficiency increases cardiac output, and clears the venous return so that blood no longer stagnates in peripheral vessels and oedema is cleared. The immediate effect of his mobilisation of fluid is an increase in urine production. Urine flow will be still further increased by the increased glomerular filtration rate and increased renal plasma flow that result from an increased cardiac output, and by a small direct action of digitalis to inhibit tubular reabsorption of sodium.

E FALSE Following the massive loss of oedema fluid described above (see D) body weight will fall.

Cardiovascular System — Cardiac glycosides: related questions 34, 35

99 Procainamide alters cardiac and particularly ventricular rate by which of the following mechanisms

    A increased excitability of the pacemaker tissue
    B increased conduction velocity in the bundle of His
    C prolongation of the effective refractory period
    D an acetycholine-like effect
    E cardiac β-blockade

A FALSE The threshold potential at which myocardial cells are stimulated is increased by procainamide so that the excitability of the muscle is depressed. Generation of impulses from both pacemaker tissue and from ectopic sources is thus reduced.

B FALSE Following procainamide, sodium entry into the cell is reduced so that the threshold potential is increased (see A), and the rate of rise of the action potential (dV/dt) is reduced. This has the effect of slowing conduction, especially through the conducting fibres of the bundle of His. The overall effect is a decrease in ventricular rate.

C TRUE During the effective refractory period (erp) the myocardial cell membrane is excitable, but impulses are not propagated. In the presence of Class I drugs (Vaughan Williams' classification of antidysrhythmic drugs), including procainamide, the duration of the action potential and of the erp are both increased. More importantly, however, the cells become refractory for a relatively greater portion of the action potential and may even remain refractory throughout the action potential. The effect is mainly on the atria, but because ectopic stimuli are reduced, ventricular rate falls.

D FALSE On the contrary, like quinidine (but to a much smaller extent) procainamide has an atropine-like action, which results in vagal block and may cause cardiac acceleration.

E FALSE Procainamide does not have β-blocking activity, its effect on cardiac function being due primarily to changes in cardiac electrical activity (see A, B and C).

100 Lignocaine

    A is a local anaesthetic
    B is usually given by mouth
    C reduces the maximum rate of depolarisation of the myocardial cell membrane
    D is used in the treatment of right heart failure (cor pulmonale)
    E has an antidysrhythmic mechanism of action similar to verapamil

---

A TRUE Lignocaine is the most widely used of the available local anaesthetics. Like other drugs of this type it blocks generation and conduction of impulses in nerves, apparently by blocking the rapid inflow of sodium ions essential for transmission of the wave of depolarisation. It has a similar action on cardiac cells, described as membrane stabilising.

B FALSE To produce its local anaesthetic action lignocaine is given by injection to allow infiltration of the area around the nerve. To treat cardiac dysrhythmia it is given either intramuscularly or intravenously. Following oral administration absorption is erratic with only about 35 per cent of the drug reaching the bloodstream.

C TRUE Lignocaine, like quinidine, reduces the maximum rate of depolarisation of the cell membrane during phase O of the action potential and increases the threshold potential. Both of these actions have the effect of reducing conduction velocity.

D FALSE Cor pumonale describes the cardiac failure which occurs secondarily to diseases of the lung such as chronic bronchitis or emphysema. The use of antidysrhythmic drugs such as lignocaine is always accompanied by a reduction in cardiac contractility which inevitably would reduce cardiac output further and make the failure worse. The reduction in contractility is regarded as a toxic effect and is due to impaired co-ordination of contractility due to depressed conduction.

E FALSE Verapamil is an antidysrhythmic drug that appears to work by blocking calcium channels in the myocardial membrane. A classification of antidysrhythmic drugs based on that of Vaughan Williams is as follows:

Class I   Membrane stabilisation
    (a) with *increased* duration of action potential, e.g. quinidine, procainamide, disopyramide
    (b) with *decreased* duration of action potential, e.g. phenytoin, mexiletine, lignocaine
Class II   Sympathetic blockade, e.g. propranolol, bretylium
Class III   Action potential prolongation, e.g. amiodarone
Class IV   Calcium entry inhibition, e.g. verapamil, prenylamine.

101 Quinidine produces which of the following effects on the heart

    A increased force of contraction
    B closing of sodium channels
    C inhibition of cell membrane ATPase
    D slowed conduction in the atrioventricular bundle
    E prolongation of the effective refractory period

A FALSE Within the normal therapeutic range quinidine does not significantly alter contractility of the heart. However, at higher doses and in damaged hearts by altering conduction and thus the synchrony of contraction it may depress contractility.

B TRUE The primary action of quinidine is thought to be on the sodium carrier mechanism to reduce entry during phase O of the action potential (see D) so that the rise time of the action potential is prolonged. It has been suggested that quinidine either reduces the 'availability' of the sodium carrier or using Vaughan Williams' model obstructs full opening of the h gate.

C FALSE Inhibition of cell membrane ATPase is the mechanism by which digitalis is thought to alter intracellular free Ca^{++} levels and thus produce its positive inotropic action. This is not an action of quinidine (see A).

D TRUE The rate of conduction of an impulse is determined primarily by the maximal rate of depolarisation (V_{max}) during phase O of the action potential (see diagram). This is dependent in turn on the membrane responsiveness to stimulation.

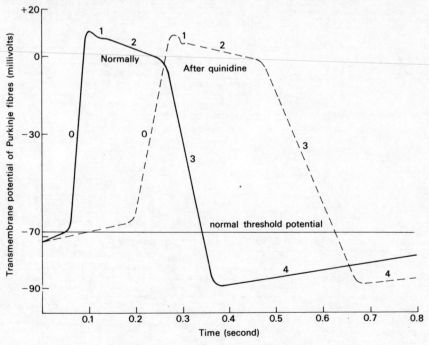

With quinidine the threshold potential is increased and the rate of rise of the action potential (dV/dt) is reduced, thus slowing conduction (see B). Reduced conduction velocity will help to interrupt re-entry of a 'circus movement', and explains part of the usefulness of quinidine. However, in incomplete heart block a reduction of atrioventricular conduction velocity may well precipitate a complete block and cause asystole.

E TRUE During the effective refractory period (erp) the myocardial cell, membrane is excitable but impulses are not propagated. For practical purposes the erp is the interval between two propagated impulses. In the presence of quinidine this interval is increased as is the total action potential duration (apd). More importantly however, the erp relative to the apd is increased by quinidine and the tissue may remain refractory after full restoration of the action potential. This is mostly a direct action of quinidine on the myocardial cells but in the atria an atropine-like action is partly responsible.

102 The antidysrhythmic drug, quinidine

A reduces the maximum rate of depolarisation of the myocardial cell membrane

B delays conduction along the bundle of His

C has a similar mode of action to verapamil

D has a similar mode of action to procainamide

E is useful in the treatment of congestive heart failure

A TRUE A reduction in the maximum rate of depolarisation of the myocardial cell membrane is one aspect of a general reduction in membrane responsiveness induced by quinidine. Its effect is primarily to reduce conduction velocity, but in turn it also reduces the refractory period.

B TRUE Conduction of electrical impulses is inhibited throughout the myocardium as described in A. Since the bundle of His is the preferred pathway of conduction between the atria and ventricles this will be inhibited most obviously.

C FALSE Using Vaughan Williams' classification for antidysrhythmic substances quinidine is a Class I drug whilst verapamil is a Class IV agent.

Class I Membrane stabilisation
   (a) with *increased* duration of action potential, e.g. quinidine, procainamide, disopyramide
   (b) with *decreased* duration of action potential, e.g. phenytoin, mexiletine, lignocaine
Class II Sympathetic blockade, e.g. propranolol, bretylium
Class III Action potential prolongation, e.g. amiodarone
Class IV Calcium entry inhibition, e.g. verapamil, prenylamine.

D TRUE Procaine is a local anaesthetic with similar membrane stabilising properties to quinidine. Procaine is rapidly metabolised in the plasma by cholinesterase and a more useful duration of action can be obtained with procainamide which is resistant to such attack.

E FALSE Myocardial contractility is impaired by quinidine and similar drugs, because contraction becomes unco-ordinated as a result of inhibited conduction. The outcome may thus be a fall in cardiac output which would exacerbate failure in congestive heart disease. Only in failure due to dysrhythmia would quinidine be beneficial.

103 The adrenergic blocker propranolol when used in the treatment of abnormal cardiac rhythms

    A acts by virtue of its antiadrenergic effects
    B acts by virtue of its membrane stabilising action
    C is helpful in the presence of heart failure
    D is useful to treat complete heart block
    E blocks β-receptors throughout the body

A TRUE Propranolol is a non-selective β-blocker which in the presence of significant sympathetic nerve activity or circulating adrenaline and noradrenaline, reduces the heart rate, prolongs atrioventricular conduction time and reduces cardiac contractility. These are all antiadrenergic actions and make it especially useful for the treatment of supraventricular tachycardias.

B FALSE Although propranolol possesses membrane stabilising (quinidine-like) activity, the doses required to produce this effect are higher than those required for β-blockade. In clinical use it would appear that the membrane stabilising effect of propranolol contributes little to the treatment of arrhythmia; some β-blockers do not have membrane stabilising activity yet are still useful agents.

C FALSE In patients in whom there are serious disturbances of cardiac rhythm, cardiac output is to some extent maintained by an adrenergically mediated increase in contractility. Use of propranolol may help to control the dysrhythmia, but may at the same time precipitate failure. Digitalis may be required to improve contractility.

D FALSE In complete heart block there is no conduction down the atrioventricular bundle and the atria and ventricles are beating independently at their intrinsic rhythms. The ventricular rate is usually between 30 to 50 beats/minute. Unless associated with failure treatment is unnecessary, but if the cardiac output falls the drop in cerebral blood flow may lead to unconsciousness. Under these circumstances a β-stimulant like isoprenaline would be required to increase the heart rate and raise cardiac output.

E TRUE Propranolol blocks both β_1 and β_2-receptors, so not only are cardiac rate and force of contraction reduced, but β-receptors in the lungs, skeletal muscle, intestine, bladder etc. are also blocked. Actions at these sites contribute to its complications and contraindications.

Cardiovascular System — Antidysrhythmic drugs: related question 72

104 5-hydroxytryptamine (5-HT)

    A is found primarily in the gastrointestinal tract
    B is metabolised by monoamine oxidase (MAO)
    C is depleted from body stores by reserpine
    D is a potent vasoconstrictor
    E has its actions antagonised by methysergide

A TRUE About 90 per cent of 5-HT in the body is found in the enterochromaffin cells of the gastrointestinal tract. In an adult this amounts to about 10 mg.

B TRUE 5-HT is a monoamine and is readily broken down by MAO to 5-hydroxyindolacetaldehyde. This is the first step in the metabolic degradation of 5-HT.

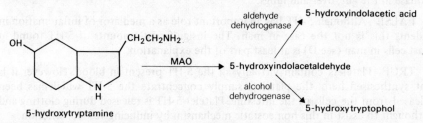

C TRUE Reserpine depletes neuronal vesicle stores of 5-HT and other amines in both the central and peripheral nervous system. It also brings about a reduction of platelet 5-HT in a similar manner, and 5-HT levels in enterochromaffin cells of the gut may be reduced to 10 per cent of their previous value.

D TRUE 5-HT is a potent vasoconstrictor, hence its other name serotonin which was given originally to the contaminating vasoconstrictor agent found in some serum samples.

E TRUE Methysergide is a 5-HT antagonist related to lysergic acid diethylamide (LSD). It may be of value in some patients with migraine, and is used to control the symptoms of carcinoid syndrome.

105 In man 5-hydroxytryptamine (5-HT) is
  A released from argentaffin cells in the gut during peristalsis
  B an important mediator of inflammation
  C found in high concentrations in platelets
  D found in high concentrations in mast cells
  E present in the diet

A TRUE There is a basal release of 5-HT from stores in the gastrointestinal chromaffin cells. This release increases during peristalsis, but the suggestion that it forms part of a physiological mechanism controlling peristalsis remains unproven. The released 5-HT is either taken up by platelets or destroyed by monoamine oxidase in the gut, liver and lungs.

B FALSE Although 5-HT has an important role as a mediator of inflammation in rodents this is not the case in man. The insignificant amounts of 5-HT found in mast cells in man (see D) is at least part of the explanation.

C TRUE Platelets contain virtually all the 5-HT present in blood. However it is not synthesised here, the platelets simply concentrate the 5-HT which has been released from the cells of the intestine. Platelet 5-HT is released during clotting and is thought to assist in this homeostatic mechansim by inducing vasoconstriction.

D FALSE Human mast cells (unlike rodent mast cells) do not normally contain 5-HT, although some mast cell tumours may.

E TRUE 5-HT is present in many fruits, e.g. bananas, pineapples, tomatoes and some shellfish, e.g. oysters, edible mussels. Nevertheless, this is probably inactivated in the liver following absorption. Body 5-HT is readily synthesised from dietary tryptophan.

106 In the aetiology of which of the following conditions in humans has 5-hydroxytryptamine (5-HT) been implicated

A migraine
B acute anaphylactic shock
C carcinoid syndrome
D allergic rhinitis (hay fever)
E hereditary angio-oedema

A TRUE In many patients who suffer from migraine there is increased urinary excretion of 5-hydroxyindolacetic acid (a metabolite of 5-HT); drugs like reserpine that release 5-HT may induce an attack; and 5-HT antagonists like methysergide have some value as prophylactics, perhaps by preventing the initial vasoconstrictor phase. Even the vasoconstrictor ergotamine has anti-5-HT activity and this property may be essential to its usefulness in the treatment of migraine.

B FALSE Acute anaphylactic shock is a Type I systemic hypersensitivity reaction which may follow injection of foreign proteins and some drugs. The features are bronchoconstriction, urticaria, pulmonary oedema, hypotension and cardiovascular collapse. They are due to mast cell degranulation following interaction of specific antigen with cell-bound (reaginic) IgE antibody on the membrane. One of the main mediators of the response is histamine. In man 5-HT is not normally present in mast cells.

C TRUE Carcinoid syndrome is a condition characterised by facial flushing, diarrhoea, bronchial asthma, and cardiac fibrosis. It is due to tumours of argentaffin tissue in the gut (particularly the appendix) which secrete large amounts of 5-HT into the circulation (although kinins and prostaglandins may also be involved). Anti-5-HT drugs may have some value in controlling attacks.

D FALSE Hay fever is a local Type I hypersensitivity reaction (see B) in which mast cell degranulation is restricted to the upper respiratory tract. Histamine is the most important mediator, and in many patients antihistamines provide effective treatment. 5-HT is not thought to be released from mast cells in man, and anti-5-HT drugs are not of value in treatment.

E TRUE Hereditary angio-oedema is a rare condition in which there is oedema, nausea, vomiting and abdominal colic. The plasma protein, complement C_1 esterase inhibitor is deficient with the result that the complement cascade and the formation of bradykinin from kallikrein are both triggered more easily. 5-HT is not apparently involved.

107 Which of the following statement is/are correct

    A cimetidine is an H_1-receptor blocker

    B the 5-hydroxytryptamine (5-HT) antagonist methysergide is used to control migraine

    C cyproheptadine is a 5-HT antagonist

    D cyproheptadine is a histamine antagonist

    E aprotinin (Trasylol) is a competitive antagonist of bradykinin

---

A FALSE Cimetidine is an H_2-receptor blocker. It will block the pharmacological actions of histamine to induce gastric acid release, to inhibit uterine contraction, and to increase heart rate. It is used clinically to treat peptic ulcers.

B TRUE In some patients following a migraine attack, there is an increased excretion of 5-HT metabolites in the urine, suggesting possible involvement of 5-HT in the aetiology of the disease. The 5-HT antagonist methysergide is also useful in some patients when given prophylactically. It is thought to prevent the vasoconstriction phase, apparently caused by 5-HT, which precedes the painful vasodilator phase.

C TRUE In addition to its antihistaminic properties (see D) cyproheptadine has equally powerful anti-5-HT action, weak anticholinergic activity and mild central depressant properties.

D TRUE The structure of cyproheptadine bears some resemblance to the phenothiazine drugs and like many of them it has potent antihistaminic properties.

E FALSE There are no clinically useful competitive antagonists of bradykinin. Aprotinin is a protease inhibitor prepared commercially from bovine lung that inhibits the action of kallikrein and hence the production of bradykinin from kininogen. It is a polypeptide with a molecular weight of around 6,500 and is sometimes used in acute pancreatitis to prevent the liberation of bradykinin by trypsin.

108 Prostaglandins (PGs)

    A are synthesised from unsaturated fatty acids
    B are stored in vesicles in a variety of cells throughout the body
    C are potent pain producing agents
    D have their action terminated by aspirin
    E modulate the activity of cyclic adenosine monophosphate (cAMP)

A TRUE 20-carbon unsaturated essential fatty acids such as arachidonic acid are the common precursors of PGs synthesised in the body. Such fatty acids are produced by lipolysis of phospholipids, triglycerides, cholesterol esters, and non-esterified fatty acids (see diagram).

B FALSE PGs are ubiquitous substances found in tissues and fluids throughout the body. However, they are synthesised and released as required — not stored.

C FALSE PGs only produce mild pain when injected intradermally in man, but smaller amounts that are without effect in their own right will markedly potentiate the pain producing effects of other mediators such as bradykinin and histamine.

D FALSE Aspirin is useful in counteracting the pathological role of PGs because it inhibits the cyclo-oxygenase enzyme responsible for their synthesis. It does not interfere with the action of PGs.

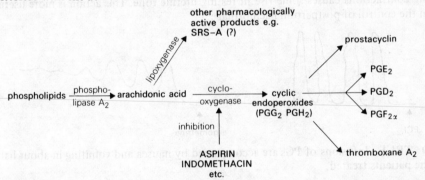

E FALSE PGs may inhibit or stimulate the activity of adenyl cyclase, depending on the particular PG and the cell type involved. Their action is described as modulatory. The effect is to increase or decrease the production of cAMP within the cell. PGs do not modify the *activity* of cAMP.

109 Prostaglandin (PG)-induced uterine contraction is

    A a clinically useful method for inducing labour
    B a useful method for producing abortion during the second trimester of pregnancy
    C similar in nature to that produced by ergometrine
    D accompanied by vomiting when given by infusion
    E characteristically accompanied by a rise in body temperature

---

A TRUE Intravenous infusion of $PGF_{2\alpha}$ and PGE_2 may be used as an alternative to oxytocin as a means of inducing labour. The type of contraction is generally indistinguishable from that produced by oxytocin. Local administration of PGs (as a pessary) may also be used. This has the added advantage of softening and ripening the cervix.

B TRUE By virtue of the powerful uterine contractions induced by PGs they have been shown to be useful in inducing abortion. The success rate is highest and the toxic effects minimal if given by intra-amniotic injection. In the first trimester of pregnancy suction curettage still remains the method of choice.

C FALSE Infusions of PGs produce sustained labour-like contraction with the uterine tone falling between each contraction. Ergometrine in addition to producing contractions causes some rise in resting uterine tone. This action is more useful in the control of postpartum haemorrhage.

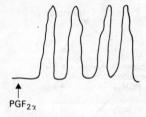

$PGF_{2\alpha}$ ergometrine

D TRUE Infusions of PGs are accompanied by nausea and vomiting in about half the patients treated.

E TRUE Prostaglandins and especially those of the E series are potent pyrogens, and a rise in body temperature commonly follows their use.

110 Bradykinin

    A contracts smooth muscle of blood vessels in the skin
    B contracts smooth muscle of the intestine
    C actions are inhibited by aprotinin
    D is stored in platelets
    E formation occurs in angio-oedema

A FALSE Bradykinin is one of the most potent vasodilators known, causing, when injected, facial flushing and a headache. It may well have a functional role as a vasodilator in the salivary glands.

B TRUE Contraction of extravascular smooth muscle is a feature of bradykinin, and the characteristically slow contraction of guinea pig ileum which it produces prompted the name bradykinin.

C FALSE There are no specific antagonists for bradykinin action. Aprotinin is a protease inhibitor prepared commercially from bovine lung. It is a polypeptide with a molecular weight of about 6,500 and inhibits proteolytic enzymes throughout the body including those responsible for the production of bradykinin. It is biologically standardised in terms of its ability to inactivate kallikrein, and is used to treat acute pancreatitis where trypsin released from the pancreas splits bradykinin from kininogen to cause cardiovascular shock.

D FALSE Platelets contain large amounts of 5-HT and heparin, but not bradykinin. Bradykinin is split from a plasma globulin precursor (bradykininogen) by the action of the proteolytic enzyme kallikrein. Bradykinin is rapidly broken down and is not stored in the body.

E TRUE The conversion of kallikreinogen to kallikrein is normally inhibited by the presence of complement C_1 esterase inhibitor in plasma. In hereditary angio-oedema there is a deficiency of this inhibitor so that kallikrein levels can rise bringing about the conversion of bradykininogen to bradykinin.

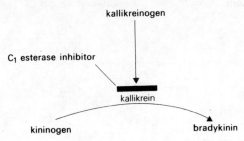

111 Bradykinin

    A gets its name from the slowing of the heart that it induces
    B is released in carcinoid syndrome
    C is found in high concentrations in mast cells
    D is removed from the circulation very slowly
    E is an important mediator of the acute inflammatory response in man

---

A FALSE Bradykinin gets its name from the characteristically slow contraction of smooth muscle of the guinea pig ileum that it produces. Because bradykinin releases catecholamines from the adrenal medulla it will, if anything, increase heart rate.

B TRUE Carcinoid syndrome is the name given to the condition characterised by facial flushing, diarrhoea, bronchoconstriction and cardiac fibrosis. It is due to the presence of argentaffin tumours in the gut that secrete 5-hydroxytryptamine and kallikrein into the circulation. The latter by releasing kinins is thought to be to a large extent responsible for the facial flushing and bronchoconstriction.

C FALSE Bradykinin is released from a plasma globulin precursor by the proteolytic action of various enzymes, particularly kallikrein. It is not stored in the body and is rapidly broken down in the circulation by kininases (see D).

D FALSE Bradykinin in the circulation has a half-life of less than 30 seconds, being destroyed by kininases present both in the plasma and bound to tissues, especially the lung.

E TRUE Bradykinin causes pain, vasodilatation, increased venular permeability and mobilisation of leucocytes — all features of the inflammatory response. However, because they are rapidly destroyed free kinins are not found in large amounts in inflammatory tissue. Nevertheless, they have been detected in animals in lymph draining from injured limbs, and from synovial fluid in patients with gout and arthritis. Increased levels of kallikrein have also been detected especially following anaphylactic reactions.

112 The synthesis of bradykinin is

    A from a plasma globulin precursor
    B activated by Factor XII (Hageman Factor)
    C inhibited by kallikrein
    D inhibited by snake venoms
    E inhibited when complement C_1 esterase inhibitor is deficient

Note:

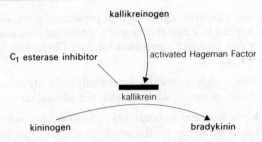

A TRUE The precursor from which bradykinin is cleaved, namely kininogen, is a plasma α_2-globulin.

B TRUE Activated Factor XII (Hageman Factor) brings about the conversion of kallikreinogen to kallikrein which is in turn responsible for the cleavage of bradykinin from kininogen. It can do this both directly or by the activation of intermediary factors such as plasmin.

C FALSE See B.

D FALSE Snake venoms contain a variety of proteolytic enzymes which are capable of cleaving bradykinin from its α_2-globulin precursor. Part of the shock reaction that follows a snake bite is due to the systemic release of bradykinin.

E FALSE Inherited deficiency of C_1 esterase inhibitor produces the rare condition known as familial angio-oedema in which there are recurrent episodes of oedema in subcutaneous tissues especially the eyelids, mouth, tongue and larynx, together with nausea, vomiting and abdominal colic. Normally C_1 esterase inhibitor not only limits the activation of the complement pathway but also inhibits the activation of kallikrein thus reducing kinin formation. When this inhibitor is deficient kinin production is more readily provoked.

113 Which of the following effects are produced by bradykinin

   A stimulation of pain fibres
   B stimulation of sympathetic ganglia
   C decrease in blood vessel permeability
   D vasoconstriction in the salivary glands
   E a rise in diastolic blood pressure

A TRUE Kinins are powerful algesic agents producing a transient but intense burning pain when applied to a blister base and a throbbing pain if injected into the hand. The action is due to direct stimulation of pain fibres, and is potentiated in the presence of prostaglandins.

B TRUE In relatively high concentrations bradykinin stimulates sympathetic ganglia and causes release of catecholamines from the adrenal medulla.

C FALSE Bradykinin increases permeability, and like 5-hydroxytryptamine and histamine, the action is primarily on the small venules to cause separation of the junctions between the endothelial cells.

D FALSE Bradykinin is a potent vasodilator and there is some evidence to suggest that it may have a functional role in mediating vasodilatation in exocrine glands including the salivary glands. In any event bradykinin does not cause vaso-constriction in these tissues.

E FALSE Because of its vasodilator action (see D) bradykinin reduces peripheral resistance producing a sharp fall in both systolic and diastolic blood pressure. This is commonly accompanied by a reflex increase in heart rate.

114 Histamine in the body

    A is synthesised by decarboxylation of histidine
    B comes mainly from intestinal bacteria
    C is stored primarily in mast cells
    D is produced in large amounts by growing cells
    E is excreted primarily unchanged

A TRUE Histidine is the major precursor of histamine in the body. Only small amounts of histamine are present in the diet and most of this is inactivated by intestinal bacteria.

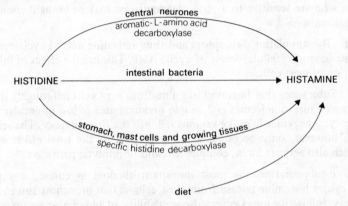

B FALSE Although histamine is produced in large amounts by intestinal flora, most is inactivated by the bacteria and little is actually absorbed. Most synthesis occurs in the tissues as a result of histidine decarboxylase activity.

C TRUE Most histamine in the body is stored in mast cells in a complex with heparin. Smaller but still substantial amounts are found in the cns, the gastrointestinal mucosa and the epidermis. The histamine synthesised at these sites tends to be released rather than stored.

D TRUE In tissues undergoing rapid growth or repair, especially fetal tissue, bone marrow and wound tissue, the production of histamine is rapid. Such tissues are said to have a high histamine-forming capacity (HFC). The histamine produced is not stored and is thought to play a role in anabolic processes.

E FALSE Only 2 to 3 per cent of histamine is excreted unchanged; the majority undergoes oxidative deamination or methylation.

115 Which of the following substances by a direct action degranulate mast cells to cause liberation of histamine and other mediators

    A aspirin
    B adrenaline
    C snake venoms
    D curare
    E morphine

A FALSE Aspirin does not bring about release of mediators from mast cells in the way that other liberators do (see below). However, in a small percentage of the population who are sensitive to aspirin, degranulation may be brought about by an indirect mechanism.

B FALSE By stimulating β-receptors and thus activating adenyl cyclase, adrenaline will increase intracellular levels of cyclic AMP. This has the effect of inhibiting degranulation of mast cells.

C TRUE Substances that liberate histamine from mast cells fall roughly into two types, complex macromolecules and simple organic bases of low molecular weight. The proteolytic enzymes in snake venoms fall into the first category. The release of histamine, however, only accounts for a small part of the total effect of these agents which also activate kinin, complement and fibrinolytic pathways.

D TRUE d-tubocurarine, the most important alkaloid in curare, is a tertiary amine. It causes histamine release from mast cells so that bronchospasm and hypotension may follow its use. Decreased coagulability of blood also occurs which is probably due to concomittant release of heparin.

E TRUE Morphine has a phenanthrene structure and can bring about histamine release from mast cells. Locally, this would produce a wheal at the site of injection, but systemically, histamine-induced bronchoconstriction added to the depressant effect of morphine on respiration, can seriously aggravate pre-existing respiratory problems, e.g. asthma.

116 The pharmacological effects of histamine include
    A gastric acid release
    B gastric pepsin release
    C contraction of smooth muscle of the intestine
    D dilatation of terminal arterioles
    E pain following intradermal injection

A TRUE In man a single dose of histamine (0.04 mg/kg subcutaneously) causes the secretion of reproducible amounts of gastric acid. At one stage this was used as a test of gastric function, having first given an H_1-antihistamine drug to reduce the cardiovascular consequences. The acid output correlates well with the parietal cell mass of the stomach. Pentagastrin is now used for this purpose.

B TRUE Histamine stimulates release of pepsin from chief (zymogenic) cells in the stomach in a similar manner to acid release from parietal cells. Both actions are blocked by the H_2-blocker, cimetidine.

C TRUE With the exception of small blood vessels (see D) histamine produces contraction of smooth muscle in most tissues throughout the body. The principal effects are bronchoconstriction and contraction of intestinal smooth muscle. The latter has long been used by pharmacologists as a technique for assaying the minute amounts of histamine in tissue fluids.

D TRUE Parenteral injection of histamine in man is characterised by dilatation of blood vessels throughout the body, but particularly in the skin of the face, neck and upper part of the body (the so-called blush area). This is often described as 'capillary dilatation', but in strict morphological terms capillaries are only a few microns in diameter and are devoid of smooth muscle. The dilatation occurs primarily in terminal arterioles.

E TRUE Whether injected into the skin, released from mast cells by drugs such as curare, or introduced inadvertently as a nettle sting, histamine produces intense itching and in high concentrations pain. It is due to stimulation of nerve endings.

117 Antihistamines like promethazine

    A produce a dry mouth
    B inhibit gastric acid secretion
    C are useful in the treatment of asthma
    D are effective in the treatment of hay fever
    E produce drowsiness

A TRUE Promethazine has some atropine-like activity which accounts for the dry mouth and blurring of vision commonly experienced during its use.

B FALSE Promethazine is an H_1-histamine antagonist and as such is without effect on gastric acid secretion which is an H_2 effect.

C FALSE Although histamine is released from mast cells in asthma and may be responsible for some of the inflammatory components of the disease, the broncho-constriction is due primarily to slow reacting substance of anaphylaxis (SRS-A) and antihistaminic drugs have proved of little value in treatment.

D TRUE Hay fever is an allergic condition in which histamine is a prominent mediator, and H_1-antagonists are an effective form of treatment. However, it should be added that drugs producing less hypnosis than promethazine are generally used, e.g. chlorpheniramine, phenindamine.

E TRUE Most antihistamines of this type are cns depressants and promethazine in particular causes drowsiness following its use. This property is used to advantage in children where it is prescribed as a combined treatment for allergic or inflammatory conditions that may prevent sleep (e.g. itching, teething).

Autacoids: related question 134

118 Gout

A is a condition in which urea crystals are deposited in the tissues
B may be treated with busulphan
C may be precipitated by diuretic therapy
D may be treated with sulphinpyrazone
E treatment with uricosurics may cause crystalluria

A FALSE Gout is a disease of uric acid metabolism characterised by high blood levels of uric acid and the deposition of crystals of monosodium urate in the tissues (tophi).

B FALSE Busulphan is an alkylating agent which because of its ability to interfere with DNA replication and hence cell division is used in the treatment of various malignant conditions. It is not used in the treatment of gout; quite the contrary, because of the rapid lysis of tissues and nucleoprotein breakdown which follows its use, it may actually induce gout.

C TRUE Chlorothiazide and related diuretics compete with uric acid for secretory transport in the kidney tubules. This causes uric acid retention, hyperuricaemia and occasionally attacks of gout.

D TRUE Sulphinpyrazone is a derivative of phenybutazone that inhibits reabsorption of uric acid by the proximal tubules of the kidney, thereby increasing uric acid excretion, a so-called uricosuric action.

E TRUE Because of the high concentration of uric acid in the tubular fluid following treatment with uricosurics, urate crystalluria may occur. A high fluid intake (3 l/day) is recommended and alkalinisation of the urine may be necessary.

119 In the treatment of gout

    A aspirin and sulphinpyrazone are the most effective combination
    B allopurinol acts by increasing uric acid excretion
    C allopurinol will inhibit the action of methotrexate
    D uricosuric drugs may cause crystalluria
    E diuretic therapy is effective

A FALSE Sulphinpyrazone is a highly effective uricosuric agent that works by inhibiting the proximal tubule reabsorption of uric acid. Aspirin in large doses ($>5g/day$) has a similar action, but in normal therapeutic amounts inhibits distal tubule secretion of uric acid, and may therefore increase blood urate levels. Whatever the dose, however, aspirin should not be given in conjunction with sulphinpyrazone, since they have a mutually antagonistic action to prevent the inhibition of urate reabsorption which they both effect at the proximal tubules.

B FALSE Uric acid is the final metabolite produced from purine metabolism. In gout there is an abnormality of this system that results in excessive blood urate levels.

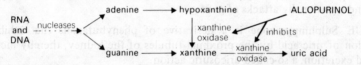

Allopurinol reduces blood urate levels by inhibiting the xanthine oxidase enzyme which converts hypoxanthine and xanthine to uric acid. Uric acid excretion therefore falls, but the excretion of both xanthine and hypoxanthine which are water soluble substances increases.

C FALSE Methotrexate is a folic acid antagonist and does not interfere with the action of allopurinol. However, another cytotoxic agent, mercaptopurine, is normally metabolised to some extent by xanthine oxidase, and inhibition of the enzyme with allopurinol will potentiate the action of this drug.

D TRUE By decreasing the proximal tubular reabsorption of uric acid, uricosuric drugs will increase the concentration of urate in the urine several fold. This may cause supersaturation, and the formation of crystals in the urine. Deposition of such crystals in the urine may be prevented by a high fluid intake (3 l/day) and alkalinisation of the urine (by giving sodium bicarbonate or potassium citrate).

E FALSE Diuretics are not useful agents in the treatment of gout, and agents like the thiazides and the loop diuretics, e.g. frusemide and ethacrynic acid, actually decrease uric acid secretion, and so may precipitate attacks of gout. Such diuretics are organic acids and are thought to prevent urate secretion by competing for the transport system.

120 Phenylbutazone

   A is a useful inhibitor of uric acid synthesis
   B is analgesic
   C can cause agranulocytosis
   D is bound to circulating plasma protein
   E is contraindicated during coumarin anticoagulant therapy

---

A FALSE Phenylbutazone is uricosuric (although the chemically related sulphin-pyrazone is better) but has no effect on uric acid synthesis.

B TRUE Phenylbutazone is a pyrazolone derivative with both anti-inflammatory and analgesic properties. It is widely used in the treatment of rheumatoid arthritis and related conditions.

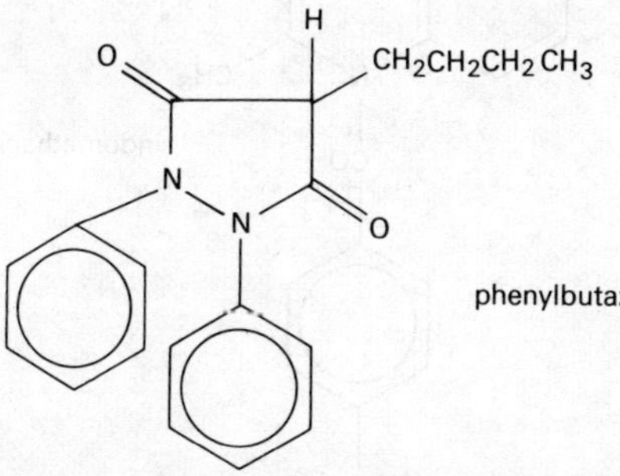

phenylbutazone

C TRUE Bone marrow depression, resulting in agranulocytosis and occasionally aplastic anaemia, is the most serious side effect of this drug. The incidence of death due to agranulocytosis is between 1 to 6/100,000 prescriptions. The mechanism is unclear but may have an immune basis.

D TRUE Only a small proportion of the plasma phenylbutazone is available to produce the pharmacological (and toxic) effects of the drug. The remainder is strongly bound to plasma albumin. This and slow metabolism by the liver mean that it has a long half-life in the body (up to 3 days) which may lead to cumulation.

E TRUE Because of its avidity for binding sites on plasma protein it will readily displace other drugs from these sites. Such an interaction occurs with the coumarin anticoagulants such as warfarin and results in increased clotting time.

121 **Chronic treatment of rheumatoid arthritis with indomethacin requires care because indomethacin**

    A is an anti-inflammatory steroid
    B causes headaches in some patients
    C inhibits the action of prostaglandins
    D causes tachycardia
    E is poorly absorbed from the gastrointestinal tract

A FALSE It is an indole acetic acid derivative with anti-inflammatory and anti-pyretic actions.

indomethacin

B TRUE Headaches and dizziness occur frequently at the outset of treatment, especially if large doses are given. In about 20 per cent of patients it may be sufficiently severe to warrant discontinuing therapy.

C FALSE Indomethacin is a potent inhibitor of prostaglandin (PG) synthesis but does not significantly alter the action of PGs. Inhibition of synthesis is thought to be the mechanism by which such non-steroidal anti-inflammatory agents produce their beneficial actions and may be responsible for some of the toxic effects, e.g. peptic ulceration.

D FALSE There have been occasional reports of oedema and hypertension, but tachycardia is not a feature of indomethacin usage.

E FALSE Indomethacin is readily absorbed from the gastrointestinal tract, peak plasma concentrations being reached in half to 2 hours, after oral administration.

122 Of the drugs used in the treatment of rheumatoid arthritis
  A indomethacin is strongly bound to plasma protein
  B a single intramuscular injection of sodium aurothiomalate is almost completely removed from the body within 48 hours
  C mefenamic acid does not demonstrate gastrointestinal toxicity
  D azathioprine is an immunosuppressant
  E prednisolone may cause adrenal insufficiency when used chronically

A TRUE Like other non-steroidal anti-inflammatory drugs, indomethacin is strongly bound to circulating albumin.

B FALSE Gold salts, like sodium aurothiomalate, are absorbed readily after intramuscular injection and become bound to plasma proteins. The gold accumulates in the body and high concentrations are found in the kidney, liver and spleen. Only 5 per cent of an injected dose is excreted within 24 hours and a further 10 per cent over the next 7 days. After a course of treatment, gold can be detected in the urine for up to 1 year.

C FALSE Nausea and dyspepsia are common gastrointestinal side effects of mefenamic acid. Ulceration of the stomach and intestinal tract with severe diarrhoea and haematemesis have also been reported but are less common.

D TRUE Azathioprine is a derivative of mercaptopurine. It is both cytotoxic and immunosuppressant.

E TRUE Chronic prednisolone administration by suppressing adrenocorticotrophic hormone (ACTH) output from the pituitary brings about adrenal atrophy. This organ is then incapable of producing glucocorticoid release in response to stress, i.e. insufficiency exists (see diagram Q233A, page 259).

123 Which of the following statements is/are correct

    A penicillamine is the drug of first choice in rheumatoid arthritis
    B aspirin will *not* prevent the progress of arthritic disease
    C prednisolone will prevent the progress of arthritic disease
    D mephenesin has useful anti-inflammatory actions
    E dextropropoxyphene produces useful inhibition of prostaglandin (PG) synthesis

---

A FALSE Although penicillamine may have a role in the treatment of rheumatoid arthritis its toxicity puts it well down the list. The risks of use are considerable and include kidney toxicity, bone marrow depression and skin rashes. In most cases aspirin remains the drug of first choice although where compliance is poor, benorylate or one of the newer agents which are administered less frequently and in smaller amounts may be more appropriate.

B TRUE Aspirin and other non-steroidal anti-inflammatory drugs will control the pain and acute exacerbations of the disease but they do not interfere fundamentally with the arthritic process.

C FALSE Anti-inflammatory steroids like prednisolone whilst powerfully anti-inflammatory do not prevent progress of arthritis in the long term and indeed by virtue of their ability to enhance weight gain, osteoporosis, and avascular bone necrosis they may further complicate treatment.

D FALSE Mephenesin is a propanediol derivative related to the tranquilliser, meprobamate. Taken orally it has some usefulness in relaxing spastic muscles by an action both on the brain and spinal cord. It is not anti-inflammatory.

E FALSE Dextropropoxyphene is related to methadone, and as such demonstrates opiate-like analgesic activity. It does not produce significant inhibition of PG synthesis.

124 Aspirin

    A reduces the raised body temperature of fever
    B reduces the normal body temperature
    C reduces the raised body temperature of heat stroke
    D antagonises the temperature elevating effect of prostaglandin E_1 (PGE$_1$)
    E inhibits the formation of endogenous leucocyte pyrogen

A TRUE Endogenous pyrogen released from leucocytes during fever acts directly on the thermoregulatory centre in the hypothalamus to increase the body temperature. This temperature elevating action of pyrogens is inhibited by salicylates including aspirin (see D).

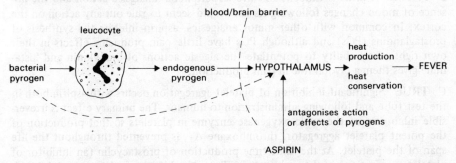

B FALSE In the absence of pyrogens, aspirin has no temperature lowering action; it is without effect on normal body temperature.

C FALSE In heat stroke the elevated temperature is due to hypothalamic malfunction and aspirin is again without effect.

D FALSE PGE$_1$ is one of the most potent pyrogens known and markedly elevates body temperature when injected into the anterior hypothalamus. Its action is not antagonised by aspirin. The action of endogenous pyrogen which is associated with a rise in cerebrospinal fluid and brain PG levels is on the other hand prevented following salicylate administration. Whether aspirin is antipyretic because it inhibits PG synthesis in the hypothalamus is, however, still controversial.

E FALSE Although the pyretic effects of endogenous leucocyte pyrogen are antagonised by aspirin most evidence suggests that the production of pyrogen and its penetration into the brain are unaffected.

125 Aspirin

   A is salicylic acid
   B produces analgesia primarily by its effect on the cortex to alter perception of pain
   C reduces platelet aggregation
   D uncouples oxidative phosphorylation
   E is excreted primarily unchanged

A FALSE Aspirin is acetylsalicyclic acid, but is readily converted in vivo to salicylic acid (see E).

B FALSE Aspirin is thought to have a 'peripheral' analgesic action and the absence of mood changes following its use would seem to rule out any action on the cortex. In common with other minor analgesics, aspirin inhibits the synthesis of prostaglandins (PGs) and although PGs have little pain producing effects in their own right, their ability to potentiate the algesic actions of bradykinin and histamine gives them a pivotal role in pain production.

C TRUE Significant inhibition of platelet aggregation occurs with aspirin both in the test tube and following administration to humans. The primary effect is irreversible inhibition of the cyclo-oxygenase enzyme in platelets so that production of the potent platelet aggregator, thromboxane A_2, is prevented throughout the life span of the platelet. At the same time production of prostacyclin (an inhibitor of platelet aggregation) in the endothelial cells of the blood vessels may be inhibited, but such cells have the ability to synthesise fresh enzyme so that prostacyclin levels are soon restored. The overall effect is one of reduced platelet aggregation and, since aggregation is often the first step in thrombosis, it has been suggested that aspirin may be beneficial in preventing further thromboembolic complications in patients who have suffered myocardial infarction. The precise value in man is still equivocal.

D TRUE Uncoupling of oxidative phosphorylation occurs with salicylates at the doses used in the treatment of rheumatoid arthritis. This causes both increased oxygen consumption and carbon dioxide production, especially in skeletal muscle. The raised blood levels of carbon dioxide lead to stimulation of respiration and together with other metabolic effects result in complex changes in the acid-base balance.

E FALSE Aspirin is readily converted by esterases in the intestinal mucosa and liver to salicylic acid and the majority of this is conjugated in the liver before excretion in the urine. Negligible amounts of aspirin will be excreted unchanged.

126 Aspirin

    A in high doses is uricosuric
    B is contraindicated during treatment of gout with uricosuric drugs
    C in toxic doses is pyretic
    D in toxic doses may produce respiratory alkalosis
    E in toxic doses may produce metabolic acidosis

A TRUE At very high doses ($>5g$/day) aspirin inhibits reabsorption of uric acid by the proximal convoluted tubules of the kidney, thus increasing its urinary excretion.

B TRUE Uricosuric drugs are effective because they inhibit the active transport system responsible for the reabsorption of uric acid in the proximal convoluted tubules of the kidney. Aspirin even at small doses will annul the uricosuric action of other drugs and is thus contraindicated.

C TRUE In high doses salicylates, including aspirin, uncouple oxidative phosphorylation in a similar manner to 2-4-dinitrophenol. Oxidative phosphorylation normally brings about the conversion of ADP to ATP. It occurs in the presence of inorganic phosphate, oxygen and specific co-enzymes, and consumes a large amount of electrical energy. Failure of this process results in dissipation of the unconsumed energy as heat with a consequent rise in body temperature.

D TRUE As a result of failure of phosphorylation pathways (see C) compensatory oxidative mechanisms bring about increased oxygen consumption and in turn increased carbon dioxide production. The carbon dioxide by a direct action on the respiratory centre stimulates respiration. Added to this, salicylates have a direct action on the medulla to increase both the rate and depth of respiration. The combined effect is to reduce plasma carbon dioxide and respiratory alkalosis ensues.

E TRUE At higher doses of salicylates than those required to produce respiratory alkalosis, and especially in children, respiratory depression occurs. Carbon dioxide production then exceeds excretion so that plasma pH decreases, i.e. respiratory acidosis exists; superimposed on this is a true metabolic acidosis due to:

1. Impaired renal excretion of phosphoric and sulphuric acid because of vasomotor depression.
2. Deranged carbohydrate metabolism with accumulation of pyruvic, lactic and acetoacetic acids in the blood.
3. The presence of salicylic and acetylsalicylic acid in the blood.

127 Because of potentially harmful effects aspirin is contraindicated in patients already receiving

    A digitalis
    B warfarin
    C barbiturates
    D antiulcer therapy
    E corticosteroids

A FALSE No therapeutically significant interactions of aspirin and digitalis occur.

B TRUE The majority of warfarin in the blood is bound to plasma protein. Such bound drug is readily displaced by aspirin increasing many times the level of free drug, and thus its anticoagulant effect.

C FALSE Although barbiturates induce liver microsomal enzymes they do not interfere with the metabolism and excretion of aspirin at therapeutic levels. Nevertheless, it has been reported that barbiturates may mask the respiratory symptoms of aspirin overdosage and may enhance its toxicity.

D TRUE Aspirin causes gastric erosions, and bleeding in many individuals, and is emphatically contraindicated in any patient suffering from peptic ulceration. The exact mechanism by which bleeding is induced is unclear, but may involve local inhibition of prostaglandin synthesis.

E FALSE There is no evidence for toxic interaction with these drugs, and many patients receiving corticosteroids for rheumatoid arthritis consume aspirin for its analgesic effect in acute episodes of the disease.

128 Paracetamol (acetaminophen)

A has clinically useful anti-inflammatory properties
B has a smaller therapeutic index than aspirin
C is chemically related to methadone
D is uricosuric
E is antitussive

A FALSE Paracetamol is only a weak inhibitor of prostaglandin (PG) synthesis, but experimentally at high doses this is sufficient to inhibit some types of experimental inflammation in animals. This is not seen clinically in man. Nevertheless paracetamol is a potent analgesic and this may be because it gains access to the nervous system and is a relatively more potent inhibitor of PG synthesis in such tissue.

B TRUE The therapeutic index is the ratio of the maximum tolerated dose of a drug to the minimum effective dose; the higher the index the safer the drug. Paracetamol has a lower index than aspirin, indicating that it has a smaller margin of safety. Death from acute paracetamol overdose is due to hepatotoxicity.

C FALSE Paracetamol is an aniline derivative.

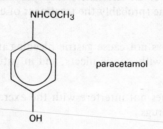

NHCOCH₃

paracetamol

OH

D FALSE Unlike aspirin, paracetamol does not have uricosuric activity. Also unlike aspirin, it may be used as an analgesic in patients receiving uricosuric therapy (e.g. sulphinpyrazone).

E FALSE Paracetamol is not antitussive; of the less powerful analgesics only opiates, like codeine, have this action.

129 **Which of the following statements relating to paracetamol (acetaminophen) is/are correct**

    A Distalgesic contains paracetamol and pentazocine

    B acute paracetamol poisoning causes hepatic damage

    C death from paracetamol poisoning may be averted by giving methionine

    D paracetamol is a useful analgesic in patients who cannot tolerate aspirin

    E paracetamol may be given in conjunction with uricosuric agents

---

A FALSE Distalgesic contains paracetamol 325 mg, and dextropropoxyphene 32.5 mg. In the UK this drug combination is currently one of the commonest causes of death from overdose.

B TRUE In adults hepatotoxicity may occur following ingestion of 10 to 15 g of paracetamol, and 25 g is likely to be fatal.

C TRUE Paracetamol is metabolised in the liver; in clinical doses it is primarily conjugated with glucuronic acid and with sulphate and only a small amount is oxidised. In overdosage, because the supply of glutathione cofactor needed for conjugation is limited, more drug is oxidised and hepatotoxic metabolites accumulate. Rapid administration of an alternative sulphydryl compound in the form of intravenous N-acetyl cysteine (probably the treatment of choice) or oral methionine may avert damage.

D TRUE Paracetamol does not cause gastric bleeding and is therefore an alternative to aspirin in patients with peptic ulcers, and in patients who are sensitive to aspirin.

E TRUE Paracetamol does not interfere with the excretion of uric acid nor the uricosuric action of other drugs.

130 Phenacetin

    A is a safer alternative to paracetamol
    B is converted in the body to paracetamol
    C has been shown to produce kidney damage
    D may cause haemolytic anaemia
    E is available to the public in self-service pharmacies

A FALSE Because of its toxicity the use of phenacetin has largely been abandoned (see C and D). Paracetamol is used in preference.

B TRUE In the normal individual 75 to 80 per cent of administered phenacetin is rapidly metabolised to paracetamol.

C TRUE Long term daily consumption of phenacetin (and possibly other analgesic preparations) has been shown to induce renal toxicity. The primary lesion is papillary necrosis with secondary interstitial nephritis. It is largely as a result of this toxicity that the availability of phenacetin in the UK has been restricted (see E), and that in some countries its use has been abandoned altogether.

D TRUE Haemolytic anaemia from phenacetin most frequently follows chronic administration, but may also occur after acute use. Haemolysis is apparently caused by metabolites that oxidise glutathione and components of the red cell membrane to shorten the erythrocyte life span. The anaemia is usually mild.

E FALSE Pure phenacetin is a 'prescription only medicine' (POM), and mixtures of phenacetin although available by prescription or on request from a pharmacist are not on display for direct sale to the public. Paracetamol should be prescribed in preference.

Anti-inflammatory Drugs and Antipyretic Analgesics: related questions 19, 25, 197, 231, 232, 233

131 In the treatment of allergic bronchial asthma

    A aminophylline acts by increasing levels of cyclic adenosine monophosphate (cAMP) in the smooth muscle of the lung

    B aminophylline stimulates the enzyme phosphodiesterase

    C cromoglycate inhibits the bronchoconstriction produced by slow reacting substance of anaphylaxis (SRS-A)

    D ephedrine is effective orally

    E 5-hydroxytryptamine (5-HT) antagonists are of value

A TRUE Aminophylline (the ethylene diamine salt of theophylline) inhibits the enzyme phosphodiesterase (see diagram opposite, Q132B, page 153). This allows cAMP to accumulate within the cells, so that the protein kinase system is activated. In the bronchiolar smooth muscle, this results in relaxation, and in the mast cells to inhibition of mediator release.

B FALSE See A.

C FALSE Disodium cromoglycate has a stabilising action on mast cells, which prevents their degranulation following the interaction between antigen and the IgE antibody on the cell surface. The drug thus provides useful prophylactic treatment of asthma, but because it does not interfere with the action of released mediators (including SRS-A) it is not of value in the treatment of an acute attack.

D TRUE Ephedrine, unlike adrenaline and isoprenaline is not destroyed by monoamine oxidase in the intestine or liver, so it is effective following oral administration. It is a mixed acting amine, but works largely by releasing noradrenaline from nerve endings.

E FALSE 5-hydroxytryptamine (5-HT), is not present in mast cells and is not thought to play a significant role in the pathogenesis of asthma. 5-HT antagonists are of no value in treatment.

132 Which of the following reduce airways resistance in *asthmatics*

   A propranolol
   B theophylline
   C aldosterone
   D isoprenaline
   E salbutamol

A FALSE   In asthmatics the full bronchoconstrictor effects caused by mediator release may be moderated by a reflex stimulation of sympathetic nerves. The amines released in this manner stimulate β-adrenoceptors on the smooth muscle of the lung to induce relaxation and on the mast cells to inhibit mediator release. If propranolol is given to such individuals (e.g. for the treatment of angina) the β-receptors in the lung are blocked, the modulating influence is removed and the patient may experience a bronchoconstrictor attack.

B TRUE   By inhibiting the action of the enzyme, phosphodiesterase, theophylline allows a build up of cyclic adenosine monophosphate (cAMP) which by an action on protein kinases causes relaxation of the smooth muscle of the bronchioles, and inhibition of the release of mediators from mast cells.

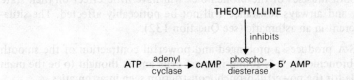

C FALSE   Aldosterone is an adrenal cortical hormone with mineralocorticoid action. It does not have anti-inflammatory activity and does not modify airways resistance in asthmatics.

D TRUE   Isoprenaline by stimulating the β-adrenoceptors in the lung activates adenyl cyclase (see B) and produces a rise in intracellular cAMP levels. This, by an action on protein kinases, causes relaxation of smooth muscle and inhibits the release of mediators from mast cells. By stimulating β-adrenoceptors in the heart, isoprenaline also causes a tachycardia.

E TRUE   Salbutamol is a selective β₂-agonist which means that it produces an essentially similar action to isoprenaline on the lung (see D) but without causing significant tachycardia (a β₁ effect).

133 Which of the following increase airways resistance in *normal man*

    A acetylcholine
    B histamine
    C propranolol
    D slow reacting substance of anaphylaxis (SRS-A)
    E promethazine

A TRUE Acetylcholine whether applied directly (e.g. by aerosol) or simply as the transmitter substance released from parasympathetic nerves supplying the lungs, produces bronchoconstriction. It does this primarily by stimulating muscarinic receptors on the smooth muscle of the bronchioles.

B TRUE Histamine has a powerful constrictor action on the smooth muscle of the bronchioles so that airways resistance increases and the FEV_1 (forced expiratory volume in 1 second) decreases. This action can be demonstrated by breathing air into which a fine spray of dilute histamine solution has been added.

C FALSE Propranolol is a β-adrenoceptor antagonist. Since the sympathetic supply to the lungs in a normal healthy man is minimal, blockade of the β_2-receptors on the smooth muscles of the bronchioles will have little effect on their state of constriction, and airways resistance will not be noticeably affected. The situation is very different in an asthmatic (see Question 132).

D TRUE SRS-A produces a prolonged and powerful contraction of the smooth muscles of the bronchioles. It is found in mast cells and is thought to be the main agent responsible for the powerful bronchoconstriction seen in asthmatics.

E FALSE Promethazine is an H_1-histamine antagonist, and as such would be expected to relieve the bronchoconstrictor effects of histamine. However, histamine is only released pathologically, i.e. following mast cell degranulation, and in normal man would not be available to stimulate receptors in the lung. Promethazine would therefore be without effect. Promethazine is also ineffective in asthmatics, but this is because it does not counteract the potent bronchoconstrictor action of SRS-A which is also released (see D).

134 In asthmatics, mast cell degranulation produced by interaction between antigen and reaginic antibody on the cell surface is inhibited by

    A acetylcholine
    B promethazine
    C cimetidine
    D disodium cromoglycate
    E salbutamol

Note: The processes of antigen induced mast cell degranulation can be depicted diagrammatically as follows:

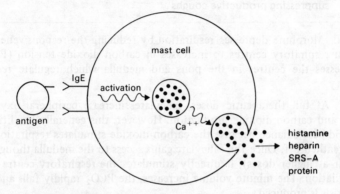

A FALSE Acetylcholine by stimulating receptors on the mast cell is thought to increase cyclic AMP levels, thus enhancing degranulation.

B FALSE Promethazine is a histamine H_1-receptor blocker which will prevent the action of released histamine but does not interfere with mast cell degranulation.

C FALSE Cimetidine is a histamine H_2-receptor blocker, the primary action of which is to inhibit gastric acid release. It does not prevent mast cell degranulation in asthmatics.

D TRUE Disodium cromoglycate has a unique mechanism of action. Whilst not interfering with antigen/antibody binding, it protects the cell from the consequences of this binding, perhaps by stabilising the cell wall. The result is that degranulation does not occur and no mediators are released. It is widely used as a prophylactic in the treatment of asthma and hay fever.

E TRUE By stimulating β_2-receptors on the mast cell, salbutamol will activate adenyl cyclase and raise intracellular levels of cyclic AMP. This will inhibit mast cell degranulation, probably by an action to reduce Ca^{++} availability.

135 Which of the following statements regarding respiratory function in man is/are true

    A morphine stimulates respiration by increasing sensitivity of the medullary centre to carbon dioxide

    B salicylates in high doses have a direct action on the respiratory centre that may result in respiratory alkalosis

    C histamine is the most important mediator of bronchoconstriction in asthmatic subjects

    D analeptic drugs in general have anticonvulsant properties

    E antitussive agents like pholcodine are potent and useful agents for suppressing productive coughs

---

A FALSE Morphine depresses respiration by reducing the responsiveness of the brain stem respiratory centres to increases in carbon dioxide tension (PCO_2). It also depresses the centres in the pons and medulla which regulate respiratory rhythmicity.

B TRUE At full therapeutic doses, salicylates increase peripheral oxygen consumption and carbon dioxide production. However, this generally has little effect on the acid-base balance because the carbon dioxide stimulates respiration, and is rapidly breathed off. Once the salicylate gains access to the medulla though (which may occur at higher doses), it directly stimulates the respiratory centre to cause hyperventilation. The minute volume increases, the PCO_2 rapidly falls and respiratory alkalosis is produced.

C FALSE Histamine is certainly released from mast cells in asthmatics, but the relative ineffectiveness of antihistaminic drugs in its treatment suggests that it has a minor role. Slow reacting substance of anaphylaxis (SRS-A) is thought to be the most important mediator of bronchoconstriction, but as yet there is no specific antagonist for this substance. Recent work has shown that SRS-A is a lipoxygenase derivative of arachidonic acid containing a dipeptide structure.

D FALSE Analeptic drugs include strychnine, nikethamide, leptazol; and without exception they are all capable of causing (not preventing) convulsions. The word analeptic comes from the Greek analeptikos meaning to restore or repair, but by usage has come to refer to the group of cns stimulant drugs that cause increased rate and depth of respiration, elevated blood pressure, a return to normal of depressed reflexes and a shortening of a period of unconsciousness. Although once widely used to treat chronic hypoxia and respiratory failure from drug overdose, their use in this manner has been thoroughly discredited.

E FALSE Pholcodine is a potent and useful antitussive agent, which, unlike morphine, is neither addictive nor constipating. It is not appropriate to suppress all types of cough and only non-productive or painful coughs should be treated. Suppression of coughing in patients with incipient respiratory failure or with excessive secretion in the lungs is harmful.

Respiratory System: related questions 47, 115, 117

136 Treatment of peptic ulcers with

    A propantheline produces H_2-receptor blockade
    B cimetidine inhibits pentagastrin-induced gastric acid secretion
    C aluminium hydroxide is contraindicated during tetracycline therapy
    D ametazole (betazole) causes reduced acid secretion
    E cholestyramine inhibits histamine-induced acid secretion

A FALSE Propantheline is primarily a muscarinic blocker, but also has significant ganglion (nicotinic) blocking activity. It reduces the output of gastric acid and slows gastric emptying, actions which facilitate the neutralisation of acid by both food and antacids. There is no evidence for blockade of H_2-receptors.

B TRUE Cimetidine is a histamine H_2-receptor antagonist. It inhibits basal and nocturnal gastric acid secretion, and that which follows pentagastrin, food and sham feeding: observations which would suggest that histamine is the final common mediator in each of these pathways.

C TRUE Tetracycline absorption is impaired by the production in the gastrointestinal tract of insoluble chelates with polyvalent cations such as Ca^{++}, Mg^{++} and Al^{+++}. Aluminium hydroxide or other antacids should not, therefore, be prescribed during tetracycline therapy.

D FALSE Ametazole is a histamine analogue with a selectivity of action towards H_2-receptors. It can be given by intramuscular injection to stimulate gastric acid secretion, and was used as a diagnostic agent for testing gastric function, but is no longer available in the UK. Pentagastrin is used instead.

E FALSE Cholestyramine is an ion exchange resin used to lower plasma cholesterol levels. It acts by binding to bile salts in the intestinal lumen so preventing their absorption via the ileum. This causes more cholesterol in the liver to be converted into bile salts and in turn lowers the total body pool. It has no value in the treatment of peptic ulcers.

137 In the intensive treatment of peptic ulcers with antacids

  A sodium bicarbonate is useful because it is rapidly absorbed into the bloodstream
  B aluminium hydroxide gel causes systemic alkalosis
  C liberation of carbon dioxide is an essential part of the action
  D magnesium-containing salts may cause diarrhoea
  E healing of the ulcers does *not* occur

A FALSE The success of any antacid depends on its ability to neutralise hydrochloric acid in the stomach, and sodium bicarbonate does this very readily. Excess bicarbonate, however, passes into the intestine where it is rapidly absorbed, and may cause alkalaemia. This is not essential to therapy and consumption of excessive bicarbonate over long periods will cause chronic alkalaemia, which is characterised by shallow breathing and attacks of cramp (tetany).

B FALSE Aluminium hydroxide gel is a mixture of oxide, hydrated oxide and carbonate of aluminium. The colloidal solution that results is not absorbed from the gastrointestinal tract and although part of its action is due to neutralisation of gastric acid, it also provides a physical gelatinous barrier between the gastric acid and the stomach mucosa.

C FALSE Carbon dioxide is only evolved as a result of acid neutralisation when using carbonate and bicarbonate salts. Contrary to popular belief, gas release and consequent belching is not an essential part of the pharmacological action.

D TRUE Magnesium oxide, and magnesium trisilicate are commonly used antacids that do not cause systemic alkalosis, nor release of carbon dioxide. The magnesium chloride which is produced, however, is a saline purgative.

E FALSE Antacids relieve ulcer symptoms, but were not thought to affect healing. Recent trials, however, using combined aluminium and magnesium antacid therapy in large doses has shown that healing of duodenal ulcers is significantly better than with a placebo and not significantly different from cimetidine therapy.

138 In the management of gastric ulcers
 A cimetidine is more effective than bed rest
 B aspirin is a good analgesic
 C corticosteroids are beneficial
 D carbenoxolone is effective
 E tobacco smoking delays healing

A FALSE A six to eight week course of treatment with cimetidine (1g/day) is effective in healing gastric ulcers in about 75 per cent of patients, but this is no better than could be achieved by strict bed rest.

B FALSE Aspirin induces gastric bleeding and is contraindicated in patients with peptic ulcers. Paracetamol is a suitable alternative.

C FALSE Corticosteroids in pharmacological amounts impair wound healing and as such should be avoided in patients with peptic ulcers.

D TRUE By increasing the secretion of mucus from goblet cells, carbenoxolone protects the ulcers from the harmful effects of gastric acid and pepsin and allows healing to take place.

E TRUE It is generally agreed that smoking delays the healing of gastric ulcers, and that patients must stop to achieve the maximum benefit from therapy. The mechanism is unclear.

139 The treatment of gastric ulcers with carbenoxolone

    A reduces gastric acid secretion
    B increases gastric emptying
    C increases secretion of mucus from goblet cells
    D prolongs the life span of gastric epithelial cells
    E may cause glucocorticoid side effects

A FALSE Carbenoxolone has no effect on either the pH or volume of acid secreted in the stomach.

B FALSE Gastric motility appears to be unaltered by the use of carbenoxolone, but the functioning of the pyloric sphincter may be more effective so that gastric emptying is if anything delayed.

C TRUE Studies both in animals and man indicate that during carbenoxolone treatment increased amounts of mucus are secreted into the stomach. It has been suggested that stimulation of goblet cell function is the method by which this occurs. The mucus is thought to protect the gastric mucosa from acid-pepsin attack (see also D).

D TRUE During carbenoxolone treatment the life span of gastric epithelial cells is prolonged by up to 50 per cent. It is thought that the increased mucus production protects particularly the immature cells developing at the base of erosions. There is also some evidence for enhanced cell proliferation during treatment.

E FALSE Liquorice addicts develop a syndrome resembling hyperaldosteronism and carbenoxolone has a similar mineralocorticoid (not glucocorticoid) effect, i.e. sodium retention and increased urinary potassium loss. This may complicate treatment by causing oedema, potassium depletion and hypertension (especially in the elderly). Thiazide diuretic therapy with potassium supplements may overcome these problems, but the obvious choice of an aldosterone antagonist such as spironolactone cannot be used because it also reduces the therapeutic action of carbenoxolone.

140 Which of the following drugs are useful in controlling motion sickness

A metoclopramide
B hyoscine
C haloperidol
D atropine
E diphenhydramine

A FALSE Although metoclopramide can be used to treat nausea and vomiting due to gastrointestinal disorders, drugs, irradiation and uraemia, it is not effective against vomiting of labyrinthine origin, such as motion sickness.

B TRUE The powerful action of hyoscine to control motion sickness was discovered in 1944 and tried out on soldiers in preparation for the Normandy landings. It is thought to act mainly on the emetic centre to prevent stimulation from the cortex and from the sensory hair cells (maculae) of the utricle and saccule. The main disadvantages are the dry mouth and drowsiness that accompany its use.

C FALSE Haloperidol has widespread actions on the cns, primarily by blocking dopamine receptors, and is useful in the treatment of psychotic conditions. It will inhibit apomorphine-induced vomiting and has been used with success to treat nausea and vomiting postoperatively, and following antineoplastic therapy. However, like chlorpromazine it is not effective against motion sickness.

D FALSE Unlike hyoscine, atropine does not have significant depressant actions on the cns, and does not possess useful antiemetic properties.

E TRUE Like other antihistamines (H$_1$-antagonists) diphenhydramine has significant depressant actions on the cns. This enables motion sickness to be controlled, but as with hyoscine drowsiness occurs.

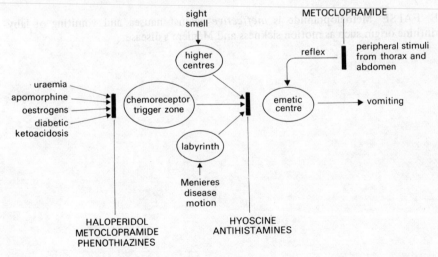

141 Metoclopramide

A may cause Parkinsonian symptoms
B is used to treat duodenal ulcers
C causes constipation
D is useful in treating vomiting following radiotherapy
E is useful in treating motion sickness

A TRUE The actions of metoclopramide on the cns are not specific for the chemoreceptor trigger zone (see D), and the appearance in some patients of extrapyramidal side effects is an indication of this. It is unwise to use it in conjunction with the phenothiazines which have a similar action.

B FALSE Metoclopramide increases gastric tone and peristalsis and the rate of gastric emptying, but not the rate of gastric acid secretion. This might be beneficial to a patient with a gastric ulcer, but is likely to be detrimental to somebody with a duodenal ulcer. This action of the drug is useful in conditions such as postoperative hypotonia of the stomach and to facilitate diagnostic barium meal examinations. The precise mechanism of action is not known.

C TRUE Although motility in the upper alimentary tract (i.e. stomach duodenum and ileum) is increased, colonic movement is unaffected or reduced, and constipation occurs in some patients.

D TRUE Metoclopramide is effective against vomiting produced by gastrointestinal disorders, drugs, uraemia and radiation, but not labyrinth disturbances (see E). Its action is in part central, due to depression of the chemoreceptor trigger zone, and in part peripheral to increase the tone of the cardiac sphincter and to promote oesophageal peristalsis thus preventing reflux (see diagram Q140, page 161).

E FALSE Metoclopramide is *ineffective* against nausea and vomiting of labyrinthine origin such as motion sickness and Ménière's disease.

142 Regarding the mechanism of action of purgatives, which of the following statements is/are correct

    A sodium sulphate is active because the $SO_4^=$ ion directly stimulates smooth muscle and peristalsis

    B the action of castor oil depends on its lubricant properties

    C liquid paraffin acts by osmotically increasing stool volume

    D compounds like phenolphthalein exert their action only on the large intestine

    E active substances from senna are absorbed in and produce their effect on the small intestine

---

A FALSE Sodium sulphate (Glauber's salt) is poorly absorbed from the gastro-intestinal tract and retains water in the bowel by an osmotic action. This promotes the formation of a bulky more fluid stool.

B FALSE Castor oil is a bland non-irritant oil that requires to be hydrolysed by lipases in the intestine before it is effective. Such metabolism produces the powerful purgative ricinoleic acid, which unlike other cathartics acts on the small intestine to produce prompt and thorough evacuation of the bowel.

C FALSE Liquid paraffin is a mixture of liquid hydrocarbons varying in absolute composition according to the source of petroleum from which it is obtained, but having a density of between 0.83 to 0.89 g/ml. The oil is indigestible, and produces an emollient or faecal-softening action, probably by retarding water absorption.

D TRUE Both phenolphthalein and bisacodyl are diphenylmethane derivatives, both of which exert their greatest effect on the large intestine. They take up to 6 hours to produce their effects, and because phenolphthalein passes through the enterohepatic cycle its action may continue for several days.

E FALSE Senna is an anthraquinone purgative, the glycosides of which are hydrolysed in the small intestine to liberate the quinones. These act on the large intestine which they reach either directly by passage through the lumen or in the blood supply following absorption in the small intestine. This circuitous route of colonic stimulation explains the delayed action of the drug.

KIDNEY — RENIN—ANGIOTENSIN—ALDOSTERONE

143 Renin

A release is promoted by a rise in renal blood flow
B release due to catecholamines is blocked by propranolol
C effects Na^+ retention by a direct action on the kidney
D acts on a plasma globulin
E is synthesised in the liver

A FALSE Either the juxtaglomerular apparatus (jga) or closely related arteriolar cells in the kidney are responsive to mechanical stress, so that as renal perfusion *falls* (due to a fall in cardiac output, or to a fall in the blood volume following haemorrhage or chronic sodium depletion) renin release occurs.

B TRUE It is generally agreed that stimulation of sympathetic nerves to the kidney and release of catecholamines into the circulation will evoke release of renin from the jga. It is also accepted that β-adrenoceptors are involved, and that propranolol will block this response. However, the site of these receptors and the possible significance of this mechanism in the hypotensive action of propranolol is more controversial.

C FALSE Renin does effect Na^+ retention by the kidney, but the mechanism is far from direct. Renin brings about release of angiotensin I from its plasma precursor. Angiotensin I is converted in the lungs to angiotensin II which in turn acts on the adrenal cortex to release aldosterone. It is the aldosterone by an action on the distal tubules of the kidney that promotes Na^+ and Cl^- reabsorption and K^+ and H^+ secretion.

D TRUE After secretion into the plasma, renin has a half-life of 15 to 30 minutes during which time it acts enzymatically on a plasma α_2-globulin (angiotensinogen) to release the decapeptide angiotensin I.

angiotensinogen (α_2-globulin)

| renin

NH_2—Asp—Arg—Val—Tyr—Ile—His—Pro—Phe—His—Leu—COOH
(angiotensin I)

E FALSE Renin is a protein of molecular weight about 40,000. It is both produced and inactivated by the kidney.

144 Which of the following is/are correct

    A The lung is the chief site for conversion of angiotensin I to angiotensin II

    B haemorrhage increases angiotensin production

    C angiotensin II is a polypeptide

    D aldosterone is synthesised from cholesterol

    E aldosterone exerts significant physiological control of glycogen metabolism

---

A TRUE The decapeptide angiotensin I is acted upon by 'converting enzyme' (a dipeptidase) which removes histidine and leucine to yield the octapeptide angiotensin II. Although converting enzymes are present in many tissues including the blood, the greatest activity is found in the lungs, and during the time it takes for the blood to traverse the lungs, in excess of 60 per cent of angiotensin I is converted to angiotensin II.

B TRUE Angiotensin I is produced from an α_2-globulin in the plasma (called angiotensinogen) by the enzymatic action of renin. Renin is released from cells of the juxtaglomerular apparatus (jga) in the kidney following stimulation of receptors (probably baroreceptors) which respond to a reduction in kidney perfusion. A rise in renin secretion and angiotensin production thus follows the fall in blood volume that occurs after haemorrhage or chronic sodium depletion.

C TRUE Angiotensin II is an octapeptide with the following structure:

$$NH_2 — Asp — Arg — Val — Tyr — Ile — His — Pro — Phe — COOH$$

D TRUE Cholesterol is the starting material for all steroidal hormones synthesised in the body; not only those synthesised in the adrenal cortex such as cortisone and aldosterone, but also the sex hormones (oestrogen, progestogen and androgens). There is overlap in the synthetic pathways.

E FALSE Comparison of the relative activities of steroids to cause sodium retention (mineralocorticoid) and deposition of glycogen in the liver (glucocorticoid) shows that aldosterone has, on a molar basis, about 30 per cent of the glucocorticoid activity of cortisol. However, the blood level of aldosterone is between one and two thousandths of that of cortisol so that in practice it has negligible action. Furthermore, the mineralocorticoid activity of aldosterone is about 10,000 times its glucocorticoid activity.

145 Which of the following statements is/are correct

A renin substrate is synthesised in the liver

B angiotensin I is converted to angiotensin II mainly in the liver

C angiotensin I possesses 50 per cent of the vasoconstrictor activity of angiotensin II

D angiotensin II releases aldosterone from the adrenal cortex

E increasing the plasma sodium concentration by an infusion of sodium chloride will stimulate aldosterone release

---

A TRUE Renin substrate (angiotensinogen) is an α_2-globulin which like most other plasma proteins is synthesised by the liver.

B FALSE The decapeptide, angiotensin I, is metabolised to the octapeptide — angiotensin II, mainly by a dipeptidase enzyme bound to the cells of the lungs. About 60 per cent of the conversion takes place after just one passage through the lungs.

C FALSE Angiotensin I has almost negligible vasoconstrictor activity, whilst angiotensin II, on a molar basis, is one of the most potent known vasoconstrictors (about 40 times the activity of noradrenaline).

D TRUE Angiotensin II acts on the zona glomerulosa of the adrenal cortex to stimulate both release and synthesis of aldosterone.

E FALSE Increasing plasma sodium concentrations by stimulating osmorecep-tors in the hypothalamus will evoke release of antidiuretic hormone (ADH) and cause water retention. The effect of this will be to increase blood volume and cardiac output, factors which would tend to improve renal perfusion and thus reduce renin release and angiotensin production, so that ultimately aldosterone release would be inhibited. Stimulation of baroreceptors in the carotid arteries would also occur so that by means of an ill-defined reflex adrenocorticotrophic hormone (ACTH) output would fall and any small facilitatory effect this substance might have on aldosterone output would be removed.

146 Which of the following effects are produced by angiotensin II

A vasoconstriction
B release of aldosterone
C diuresis by a direct action on the kidney tubules
D inhibition of adrenocorticotrophic hormone (ACTH) release by an action on the pituitary
E α-receptor stimulation

A TRUE The octapeptide angiotensin II is, on a molar basis, by far the most potent pressor agent known. It produces powerful vasoconstriction, primarily in the arterioles of skin, splanchnic regions and kidney, so that blood flow to these areas falls sharply. The action is short-lived (the half-life is less than 1 minute) because angiotensin II is metabolised by tissue-bound peptidases. Angiotensin is available as an amide for clinical use in hypotensive states.

B TRUE Angiotensin II has a direct action on the zona glomerulosa of the adrenal cortex to stimulate synthesis and release of aldosterone. They are only very limited stores of new steroid in the adrenal cortex and increased release is synonymous with increased production. The exact mechanism is unclear, but requires Ca^{++}, is accompanied by a rise in cyclic AMP (cAMP) levels, and is inhibited by puromycin.

C FALSE In addition to its indirect action via aldosterone to cause Na^+ retention and antidiuresis (see B), angiotensin does have an action on the kidney which may cause either diuresis or antidiuresis. However, this is not a direct action but is due to changes in renal blood flow and glomerular filtration rate.

D FALSE Angiotensin acts on the adrenal cortex to effect release of aldosterone (see C) but there is no evidence of an action on the pituitary to modify ACTH output.

E FALSE Although angiotensin produces powerful vasoconstriction (see A), the receptors involved are distinct from those for biogenic amines and other peptides. There is, nevertheless, some evidence that angiotensin facilitates transmitter release from sympathetic neurones, and perhaps also increases the responsiveness of the innervated organ to noradrenaline stimulation.

147 Aldosterone

    A action on the kidney is blocked competitively by triamterene
    B secretion is indirectly controlled by renin release from the kidney
    C secretion leads to K^+ retention by the renal tubules
    D secretion is increased by infusions of isotonic sodium chloride
    E is synthesised in the adrenal gland

A FALSE Aldosterone acts on the distal tubules of the kidney to cause Na^+ and Cl^- reabsorption and K^+ and H^+ secretion (see C). Triamterene acts on the distal tubules to increase Na^+, Cl^- and HCO_3^- loss whilst conserving K^+ and H^+ and, because of this apparently opposite action, it was originally thought to act by antagonising aldosterone. However, its action persists in adrenalectomised animals and in the presence of aldosterone antagonists.

B TRUE Aldosterone release from the adrenal cortex is effected by renin by means of the following series of events.

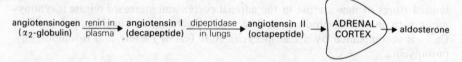

C FALSE Aldosterone is known as the 'sodium retaining factor' of the body, because of its action on the distal tubules of the kidney to promote Na^+ and Cl^- reabsorption. At the same time it also facilitates K^+ and H^+ excretion because these ions are normally exchanged for Na^+ and Cl^-.

D FALSE An infusion of isotonic sodium chloride solution by increasing blood volume will increase blood pressure. 'Volume' receptors in the carotid arteries and in the juxtaglomerular apparatus (jga) of the kidney will detect this and the effect will be a *reduction* in aldosterone output. The most important system is the jga which mediates a reduction in the output of renin (see B). The carotid artery receptors seem to be involved only if blood volume is low. An *increase* in aldosterone release occurs either as a result of reflex sympathetic vasoconstriction (which causes renin release by the kidney) or by release of adrenocorticotrophic hormone (ACTH) which has some ability to evoke aldosterone release directly. There is also evidence that low sodium and elevated potassium can evoke the release of aldosterone directly.

E TRUE Aldosterone is synthesised from cholesterol in the zona glomerulosa of the adrenal cortex. The stores of aldosterone are limited and stimuli for aldosterone secretion also cause increased synthesis.

148 Antidiuretic hormone (ADH: vasopressin)

A is secreted when plasma osmolality increases
B is synthesised in the posterior pituitary
C plays an important role in normal blood pressure control
D is useful in the treatment of nephrogenic diabetes insipidus
E acts mainly on the proximal convoluted tubule

A **TRUE** Secretion of ADH is dependent upon the osmolality of the extracellular fluid (ecf): perfusion of the internal carotid artery with solutions of sodium chloride in which osmolality has been increased only 1 to 2 per cent above the plasma value are sufficient to induce ADH release and elicit an antidiuresis. The osmoreceptors are in the region of the supraoptic nuclei in the hypothalamus.

B **FALSE** Although released from the posterior lobe of the pituitary, vasopressin is actually synthesised in the perikaryon of nerve cells composing the supraoptic and paraventricular nuclei of the hypothalamus. Vasopressin, in combination with protein carrier molecules known as neurophysins, travels down the axons to the cells of the posterior pituitary where it is stored and released. Oxytocin is synthesised and stored in a similar fashion.

C **FALSE** As the name implies vasopressin, if used in pharmacological amounts, will elevate the blood pressure. It does this by producing vasoconstriction of arteriolar smooth muscle. Physiologically, however, the role of vasopressin is limited to the conservation of body water and it is not important in the control of blood pressure. A fall in blood volume (e.g. acute haemorrhage) is thought to stimulate stretch receptors in the left atrium to evoke reflex release of vasopressin and thus induce antidiuresis.

D **FALSE** Nephrogenic diabetes insipidus refers to an inherited abnormality in which the renal tubules are unresponsive to circulating or administered ADH. True diabetes insipidus in which the pituitary has been destroyed by disease can of course be controlled by giving ADH.

E **FALSE** ADH increases the permeability of the renal collecting ducts so that as the urine passes towards the cortex, where the osmotic gradient between the peritubular fluid and collecting ducts increases, water will pass out of the tubules and the urine will become more concentrated.

149 Which of the following is/are correct

    A carbonic anhydrase inhibition in the kidney causes increased bicarbonate loss in the urine

    B mercurial diuretics produce an alkalosis

    C potassium retention may be a problem during treatment with amiloride

    D mannitol directly inhibits distal tubular sodium reabsorption

    E ethacrynic acid produces only mild potassium loss in the urine and may even lead to hyperkalaemia

---

A TRUE The carbonic anhydrase enzyme catalyses the production of carbonic acid by renal nephron cells. This provides H^+ for exchange with Na^+ in the tubular lumen, the Na^+ moving into the blood as sodium bicarbonate and thus maintaining the alkali reserve. The H^+ ions in the tubular lumen combine with bicarbonate (which has entered by filtration at the glomerulus) to form carbonic acid which as carbon dioxide and water is reabsorbed. In the presence of a carbonic anhydrase inhibitor, H^+ is not available, and the bicarbonate remains in the lumen to be excreted. The loss of this bicarbonate from the body causes acidosis.

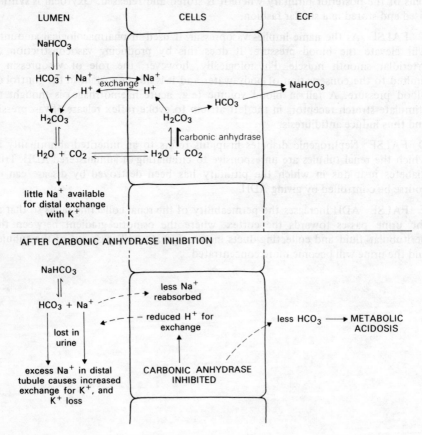

B TRUE Mercurial diuretics are concentrated in the kidney, where they produce diuresis by chelating sulphydryl groups of the enzymes and transport mechanisms involved in Na^+ absorption, mainly in the ascending limb of the loop of Henlé. The drugs are effective in acid urine (which is necessary to liberate the mercuric ion), and lose their effectiveness if the urine becomes alkaline. However, this is precisely what happens because the loss of sodium without loss of bicarbonate (they do not inhibit carbonic anhydrase) disturbs the bicarbonate buffer system.

$$H_2CO_3 + NaHCO_3 \rightleftharpoons 2HCO_3^- + H^+ + Na^+$$

$$\underbrace{H_2CO_3}$$

lost in
urine

As sodium bicarbonate in the blood dissociates and sodium is removed the bicarbonate combines with H^+ ions to form the weak (and largely undissociated) carbonic acid. Alkalosis results from this removal of H^+ ions. The effectiveness of mercurial diuretics may be restored by administration of ammonium chloride.

C TRUE Amiloride acts on the distal tubules of the kidney to increase Na^+, Cl^- and HCO_3^- loss and to conserve K^+. Although this is an action similar to the aldosterone antagonist spironolactone, it occurs in the absence of aldosterone. The potassium-sparing effect may lead to hyperkalaemia and for this reason it should not be given with other potassium-sparing agents or in renal insufficiency, but rather as an adjunct to potassium-losing diuretics. The rise in plasma potassium may cause muscle weakness, irregularity of the pulse and the danger of cardiac arrest.

D FALSE Like other osmotic diuretics, mannitol is administered intravenously, and enters the tubules by filtration at the glomerulus. It is not reabsorbed and because of its high osmotic pressure, the sodium reabsorption which occurs in the proximal tubule is not accompanied by the usual amount of water. This ensures that the tubular fluid remains iso-osmotic with plasma. Mannitol does not have a direct action on the distal tubules, and any small change in function which occurs there is a result of proximal changes in the urine composition.

E FALSE The main action of ethacrynic acid is on the loop of Henlé and the proximal part of the distal tubule to impair the concentrating mechanism. It does not inhibit carbonic anhydrase, but the high concentration of Na^+ in the tubules and the fast flow of urine mean that the Na^+-K^+ exchange in the distal tubule is enhanced and significant potassium loss occurs.

171

150 Which of the following statements about diuretics is/are correct

A frusemide has its primary action on the loop of Henlé, and gives a diuretic effect within 30 minutes of oral administration

B acetazolamide causes a self-limiting metabolic alkalosis

C ethacrynic acid is thought to act by binding to SH-groups

D mercurial diuretics are thought to act by binding to SH-groups

E the diuretic effect of triamterene is due to inhibition of antidiuretic hormone (ADH) release

---

A TRUE Frusemide is a thiazide derivative and as such it has some action on the distal tubule. It also inhibits carbonic anhydrase which means a small effect throughout the length of the tubule, but the main action is on the ascending limb of the loop of Henlé to impair Na^+ and Cl^- absorption and thus reduce the effectiveness of the counter-current multiplier. The action is sufficient to produce a potent diuresis within 30 minutes of an oral dose.

B FALSE Carbonic anhydrase inhibitors like acetazolamide inhibit the production of H^+ throughout the nephron. Such H^+ normally exchanges with Na^+ in the

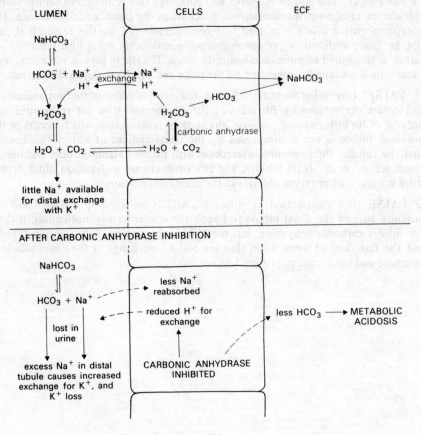

tubule, so that Na^+ excretion is effectively increased. Bicarbonate excretion also increases and because more Na^+ and less H^+ is available for exchange in the distal tubules, K^+ excretion is enhanced.

Loss of the HCO_3^- causes a *metabolic acidosis,* but this in turn reduces the efficacy of the drug because as the plasma bicarbonate falls so the amount of filtered bicarbonate is reduced. Such small amounts can be reabsorbed without the aid of carbonic anhydrase, so that no further interference with Na^+ reabsorption occurs, i.e. the action is self-limiting.

C TRUE Ethacrynic acid was developed as an agent that would bind to -SH groups and there is ample evidence that this is the case. It is thought that binding to such groups on the enzymes responsible for active transport of Na^+ in the kidney tubules is the mechanism by which it causes diuresis. Since mercurials have a similar mode of action (see D) these two diuretics are not additive. However, ethacrynic acid has a more selective action on the loop of Henlé and is consequently more potent.

D TRUE Mercurial diuretics have the general structure $X\text{-}CH_2\text{-}Hg^+$ and in acid media the $CH_2\text{-}Hg^+$ bond is broken to release the mercuric ion. It is thought that this then binds to sulphydryl-containing enzymes and/or transporting proteins in the renal tubules concerned with sodium reabsorption. The main action is on the ascending loop of Henlé. Mercurials cause alkalosis and since an acid medium is required to liberate the mercuric ion the action of the drug is self-limiting.

E FALSE Triamterene acts on the same portion of the distal tubule as spirono-lactone to increase Na^+, Cl^- and HCO_3^- loss and to conserve K^+, but unlike spironolactone it is not an aldosterone antagonist. Triamterene does not interfere with the action of ADH which acts on the collecting ducts to increase their permeability to water.

151 Thiazide diuretics

  A may precipitate gout
  B are useful in the treatment of hypertension
  C may precipitate diabetes mellitus
  D inhibit carbonic anhydrase
  E inhibit sodium reabsorption in the distal convoluted tubules

---

A TRUE Plasma uric acid levels are frequently raised in patients treated with thiazides because such diuretics compete with the transport system for urate excretion in the distal tubules. In susceptible individuals this may lead to attacks of gout.

B TRUE Thiazide diuretics provide an effective treatment for mild hypertension, and although their initial efficacy may be ascribed to the reduction in blood volume which occurs following diuresis, it is clear that this is not the complete explanation, in that they continue to be hypotensive after the blood volume has returned to normal. An action to relax peripheral arterioles and to reduce their sensitivity to vasoconstrictor agents seems to be a more important mechanism.

C TRUE Hyperglycaemia is a complication of thiazide usage, which may reveal latent diabetes mellitus in susceptible individuals and upset treatment in stabilised diabetics. Decreased insulin release from the pancreas, and inhibited peripheral glucose utilisation are suggested mechanisms.

D TRUE Related to the sulphonamide class of carbonic anhydrase inhibitors, the thiazides were first investigated as agents which might have a similar action; and although the majority of their diuretic action is due to another action (inhibition of tubular Na^+ reabsorption $-$ see E), in full therapeutic doses they significantly inhibit carbonic anhydrase.

E TRUE The main action of the thiazides is to inhibit active chloride transport and thus Na^+ reabsorption in both the cortical part of the loop of Henlé and in the proximal part of the distal tubule. The increased Na^+ in the tubules (and reduced availability of H^+ because of carbonic anhydrase inhibition) means that K^+ exchange increases and clinically significant potassium depletion also occurs.

152 The diuretic chlorothiazide

A is effective orally
B causes potassium retention
C antagonises the action of digitalis
D can aggravate diabetes mellitus
E accelerates both sodium *and* chloride loss

A TRUE Chlorothiazide is effective orally, but it is water soluble and absorption from the gastrointestinal tract is poor so that a dose of 0.5 to 2.0 g/day is required for useful diuresis. It is mainly used in conjunction with other diuretics.

B FALSE Because Na^+ reabsorption is inhibited (see E), excess of this ion reaches the distal tubules, which means that greater exchange for K^+ will occur and potassium excretion is enhanced. This is aggravated by reduced availability of intracellular H^+ (due to inhibition of carbonic anhydrase) which would normally also exchange with Na^+. Potassium supplements may be necessary.

C FALSE Digitalis inhibits the Na-K^+ membrane ATPase of the myocardial cells, and at least part of its beneficial action is due to a fall in intracellular K^+ levels. If the plasma K^+ levels are lower than normal (as produced by chlorothiazide – see B), K^+ moves down the concentration gradient more easily, the transmembrane potential is reduced, and the digitalis action is potentiated. Since digitalis has a low therapeutic ratio, this readily leads to toxicity.

D TRUE Thiazide diuretics may induce hyperglycaemia but the mechanism is unclear and may involve inhibition of insulin release and/or inhibition of peripheral glucose utilisation. Whatever the cause, it will aggravate pre-existing diabetes.

E TRUE The main sites of action of chlorothiazide are the cortical part of the loop of Henlé and the proximal part of the distal tubule. Its action is primarily to inhibit active chloride transport and thus decrease the reabsorption of Na^+, but because it also inhibits carbonic anhydrase the Na^+ is accompanied by Cl^- and HCO_3^-.

153 Organic mercurial diuretics (e.g. mersalyl) can produce

    A water loss
    B sodium loss
    C bicarbonate loss
    D chloride loss
    E metabolic alkalosis

A TRUE Water absorption in the renal tubules is diminished because the ions retained within the tubules (see B and D) act as osmotic diuretics.

B TRUE The primary action of organic mercurial diuretics is to inhibit the transport systems involved in Na^+ reabsorption. This occurs to some extent in the proximal convoluted tubule, but primarily in the ascending limb of the loop of Henlé.

C FALSE Mercurial diuretics do not inhibit carbonic anhydrase and bicarbonate loss does not occur. In fact the loss of Na^+ without HCO_3^- is the cause of the disturbance to the bicarbonate buffer system that eventually leads to alkalosis (see E).

D TRUE Chloride loss is secondary to sodium, reabsorption being impaired by electrostatic attraction of this ion to the sodium in the tubular lumen.

E TRUE Sodium bicarbonate in the blood dissociates to give Na^+ and HCO_3^-. These ions enter the renal tubules from the glomerulus and would normally be reabsorbed. However, because Na^+ reabsorption is impaired (see B), further dissociation takes place and the HCO_3^- combines with H^+ ions (provided by the carbonic anhydrase reaction, which is not inhibited) to form the weak and largely undissociated carbonic acid. This loss of H^+ from the body effects an alkalosis which, because liberation of the mercuric ion from the diuretic requires an acid environment, limits the action of the drug (see equation, Q149B, page 171).

154 Which of the following substances promote a loss of potassium from the body

    A spironolactone
    B triamterene
    C aldosterone
    D frusemide
    E carbenoxolone

A FALSE Spironolactone is an aldosterone antagonist and so will produce the opposite effects to aldosterone (see C) namely Na^+ loss and K^+ retention. In the absence of aldosterone secretion, it will have no effect, but in the presence of chronic oedema where aldosterone levels are high it produces a clinically useful diuresis.

B FALSE Once thought to be an aldosterone antagonist, triamterene has a similar action to spironolactone. However, it is effective in the absence of aldosterone (e.g. in adrenalectomised animals), and is now known to have a direct action on the distal tubule to inhibit Na^+ reabsorption and as a consequence to reduce the secretion of potassium.

C TRUE Aldosterone acts throughout the body to stimulate the sodium pump so increasing the passage of ions across membranes. This effect is most apparent in the distal tubules of the kidney where it causes Na^+, Cl^- and HCO_3^- to be retained and allows K^+ and H^+ to be lost. This occurs in primary hyperaldosteronism (Conn's syndrome), a disease which is characterised by hypertension, hypokalaemia, metabolic alkalosis, polyuria and periodic paralysis and paraesthesias.

D TRUE Frusemide is a thiazide derivative having its main action on the ascending limb of the loop of Henlé to impede Na^+ and Cl^- reabsorption and thus the efficacy of the counter-current multiplier system. The resulting copious urine flow means that Na^+-K^+ exchange mechanisms in the distal tubules are relatively ineffective and a large loss of potassium occurs. The commonest adverse effects of frusemide (i.e. muscle weakness, constipation and anorexia) are due to hypokalaemia and inadequate supplementation.

E TRUE Carbenoxolone is a liquorice derivative that is used for the treatment of peptic ulcers. Liquorice addicts may develop a syndrome resembling hyperaldosteronism (see C) in which hypokalaemia and increased urinary loss of potassium occur. A similar effect may be seen with carbenoxolone. The precise mechanism is unclear, but is partly due to potentiation of aldosterone action, and partly a direct action on distal tubules which can be blocked by spironolactone (see A).

155 Excessive *loss* of potassium is undesirable because it may produce

    A intestinal ulceration
    B intestinal haemorrhage
    C intestinal stasis
    D cardiac arrest
    E decreased response to cardiac glycosides

Note: 98 per cent of body K^+ is intracellular, but loss of around 500 mEq (about a seventh of the total) must occur before any measurable change in extracellular K^+ level is apparent. By this stage depletion is severe and hyperpolarisation of excitable membranes occurs.

A FALSE Small bowel ulceration may occur, not during hypokalaemia, but when potassium is administered orally in large amounts to treat it. The risk can be reduced by using formulations in which small amounts of K^+ are released slowly into the gastrointestinal tract, i.e. effervescent and wax or resin bound preparations.

B FALSE Some degree of haemorrhage may be associated with the ulceration caused by high potassium concentrations in the gastrointestinal tract following supplementation (see A), but potassium depletion per se does not cause intestinal haemorrhage.

C TRUE As a result of the hyperpolarisation caused by depletion (see Note) depolarisation of intestinal smooth muscle occurs less readily. This has the effect of causing muscle relaxation, intestinal stasis and constipation.

D TRUE Excessive potassium depletion causes hyperpolarisation of cardiac cells (see Note). This may lead in turn to reduced contractility, depression of the ST segment and of the T wave of the ecg, and a fall in cardiac output. If depletion is severe, this may lead ultimately to cardiac arrest. It should be noted, however, that potassium in excess, by increasing cardiac excitability, can also lead to arrest.

E FALSE The beneficial action of cardiac glycosides is accompanied by inhibition of Na^+-K^+ membrane ATPase and an increased loss of potassium from cardiac cells. When hypokalaemia occurs, the cardiac glycosides demonstrate increased efficacy and toxicity. This may be due to additional loss of potassium from the cells as a result of the increased concentration gradient, or because extracellular potassium normally inhibits glycoside binding, and additional drug now attaches to the myocardial cells.

156 Spironolactone in man

    A is a weaker diuretic than chlorothiazide
    B is a non-competitive aldosterone antagonist
    C must be given with potassium supplements
    D has a slow but prolonged action
    E may precipitate diabetes mellitus

A TRUE Since spironolactone is a competitive antagonist of aldosterone, its action is limited by the levels of circulating aldosterone and the maximal effect that aldosterone is capable of achieving. This is seem most clearly in the total absence of aldosterone (produced by removal of the adrenal cortices) where only 1 to 3 per cent of the Na^+ filtered by the glomerulus is lost from the body. Chlorothiazide on the other hand, by inhibiting the important sodium reabsorption mechanisms in the cortical part of the loop of Henlé and the distal tubule produces a greater diuresis (up to 8 per cent of filtered Na^+).

B FALSE Spironolactone is a competitive antagonist of aldosterone, and is only effective in the presence of circulating hormone (see A). Its action is the reverse of aldosterone, namely to produce Na^+, Cl^- and HCO_3^- excretion and K^+ and H^+ retention.

C FALSE Since K^+ excretion is reduced (see B) potassium supplements are unnecessary.

D TRUE The maximum response is attained after about 3 days of treatment and effectiveness continues for 2 to 3 days after stopping therapy.

E FALSE Precipitation of diabetes mellitus is a hazard of thiazide therapy due to hyperglycaemia induced by these drugs; spironolactone does not have this effect.

157 Frusemide

A is a weaker diuretic than chlorothiazide
B has its main effect on the descending loop of Henlé
C is short acting
D is effective orally
E does *not* interfere with digitalis therapy

A FALSE Frusemide is one of the 'high-ceiling' diuretics which produce a far greater peak diuresis than other agents. The extent and rapidity of action, e.g. 2 litres of urine in 90 minutes, make it ideal for the relief of pulmonary oedema in acute heart failure. Such efficacy can, however, constitute a disadvantage in that dehydration occurs.

B FALSE Frusemide like other thiazide derivatives inhibits the sodium pump throughout the nephron, but its main action is on the *ascending* loop of Henlé to impair Na^+ and Cl^- absorption. This reduces the efficacy of the counter-current multiplier system and results in a massive urine flow.

C TRUE If given orally frusemide is effective within 30 minutes and lasts for about 4 hours. If given intravenously it produces copious diuresis within 5 minutes lasting for about 2 hours.

D TRUE See C.

E FALSE Potassium lost in the urine is secreted from the distal tubule in exchange for sodium, and by virtue of the extremely rapid urine flow produced by frusemide, K^+ loss is considerable. This in turn causes hypokalaemia which enhances K^+ efflux from cardiac cells, reduces the transmembrane potential and enhances glycoside binding to cardiac cells. All of these effects potentiate the pharmacological and toxic actions of digitalis.

158 Which of the following statements about drug modification of kidney function is/are true

    A dopamine increases glomerular filtration rate
    B nephrogenic diabetes insipidus responds to antidiuretic hormone (ADH) nasal spray
    C xanthine diuretics act mainly by antagonising the action of ADH on the kidney tubules
    D osmotic diuretics act primarily by raising blood osmolality and thus inhibiting ADH release
    E probenecid has an antidiuretic action on the kidney

A TRUE In the treatment of cardiogenic shock a good indicator of cardiovascular status is the amount of urine produced per hour, a fall in urine production being indicative of a reduced cardiac output and peripheral vasoconstriction. Dopamine is a useful drug under these circumstances because it has an inotropic action on the heart and at the same time by stimulating dopaminergic receptors produces vasodilatation of the renal arterioles. The effect of this is to increase the glomerular filtration rate.

B FALSE Nephrogenic diabetes insipidus is an inherited condition in which the collecting ducts show an insensitivity to the permeability-increasing effects of ADH.

C FALSE There are no diuretics in clinical use that work by antagonising the action of ADH on the kidney. This is not surprising in that conditions of overhydration in which diuretic therapy would be appropriate, such as congestive heart failure and pulmonary oedema, would cause minimal secretion of ADH and therefore reduce the usefulness of an antagonist. The xanthines are not powerful diuretics and act mainly by increasing glomerular filtration rate.

D FALSE Osmotic diuretics are filtered by the glomerulus and enter the renal tubules where they exert a considerable osmotic pressure. As sodium is reabsorbed by the proximal tubules, it is not accompanied by the usual quantity of water which remains in the tubules to maintain the osmotic pressure of the tubular fluid at a similar level to that of plasma. This fluid is excreted, and once a high urine flow is established sodium reabsorption also becomes impaired and is excreted. A rise in blood osmolality will also occur, but by stimulating receptors in the hypothalamus, ADH release will occur and an antidiuretic effect will be induced. This will tend to reduce the efficacy of the osmotic diuretics.

E FALSE Probenecid competitively inhibits the renal tubular transport of organic acids, and can be used equally well to inhibit the tubular secretion of penicillin or the tubular reabsorption of uric acid. It does not markedly alter total urine production and in the treatment of gout a high fluid intake is advisable to prevent the formation of uric acid crystals in the urine.

Kidney — Diuretics: related questions 19, 20, 31, 32, 88

159 Within the central nervous system which of the following are inhibitory transmitters

    A glutamate
    B glutamine
    C dopamine
    D gamma-amino-butyric acid (GABA)
    E aspartate

Note: Inhibitory transmitters are substances which when released from neurones in the cns attach to receptors on the postsynaptic membrane to bring about hyperpolarisation, reduced sensitivity to stimuli and a reduced rate of firing of that neurone.

A FALSE Glutamate is found in the cns mainly in the spinal cord, and there is some evidence that it has a role as an excitatory transmitter at this site, but there is no specific antagonist to its action and its precise function remains to be established. It is also a precursor in the synthesis of GABA (see D).

B FALSE Glutamine is a metabolic derivative of ammonia and glutamic acid, and serves as a donor of amino groups in the synthesis of important compounds such as amino sugars and purine bases. It also acts as a transport system for ammonia to the kidney, but it is not thought to be a neurotransmitter.

C TRUE Dopamine is an important inhibitory transmitter. The dopaminergic systems are confined mainly but not exclusively to the mid-brain. Dopaminergic neurones are found particularly in the substantia nigra, terminating in the corpus striatum and globus pallidus. Dopamine has an important role in Parkinson's disease, schizophrenia, acromegaly and in conditions associated with excessive prolactin secretion.

D TRUE It is estimated that the two inhibitory transmitters GABA and glycine together account for about half the synapses in the cns. GABA is found mainly in the cerebral cortex, but also in the spinal cord. There is some evidence to suggest that deficiency in the GABA system underlies diseases causing choreic movements, e.g. Huntington's chorea.

E FALSE There is some evidence that aspartate is an excitatory transmitter primarily in the spinal cord.

160 Gamma-amino-butyric acid (GABA)

A is an excitatory transmitter in the cns
B increases chloride permeability in neurones
C acts on postsynaptic membranes
D has its action terminated by re-uptake into axons
E has its action blocked selectively by strychnine

A FALSE GABA hyperpolarises most central neurones, an action which reduces their rate of firing. It is, therefore, described as an inhibitory transmitter.

B TRUE GABA causes hyperpolarisation by increasing chloride conductance due to a selective change in permeability.

C TRUE The action of GABA is to reduce the rate of firing of postsynaptic neurones mainly in the cerebral cortex, where it is most widely distributed, but also in the spinal cord.

D TRUE The action of GABA is limited by a sodium-dependent uptake process into nerve and glial cells.

E FALSE Strychnine is an antagonist of another inhibitory transmitter, glycine, but does not block GABA. The actions of GABA are inhibited by the poison bicuculine which produces an overall increase in brain electrical activity and may induce convulsions.

161 Depletion of dopamine in the brain

    A may induce epilepsy

    B may cause lactation

    C may be induced with reserpine

    D may be induced with chlorpromazine

    E is an essential part of the action of lithium

A FALSE Epilepsy is the result of abnormal electrical discharge in the brain and although the reasons for this in man are not known, convulsions can be induced in animals by drugs that potentiate the action of noradrenaline and dopamine, e.g. cocaine, amphetamine. Depletion of dopamine would in these circumstances have the opposite effect.

B TRUE Galactorrhoea and some forms of infertility may be ascribed to excessive circulating levels of prolactin. The hypothalamic inhibitory factor which normally limits the secretion of prolactin from the pituitary is almost certainly dopamine, so that depletion of dopamine in the hypothalamus may cause lactation. This is seen as a side effect of drugs which block dopamine receptors (e.g. haloperidol) or which deplete brain amine levels (e.g. reserpine).

C TRUE Reserpine acts on 'aminergic' neurones in both the sympathetic and central nervous systems to deplete stores of amine from the granular binding sites of the dense core vesicles. Centrally, it has powerful sedative actions, probably due to depletion of noradrenaline, 5-hydroxytryptamine and dopamine from the neurones. Dopamine depletion also leads to the production of Parkinsonian side effects.

D FALSE The antipsychotic drug chlorpromazine has a multitude of actions on the cns, but most important amongst these, and probably the mechanism by which it is effective in schizophrenia, is its ability to block dopamine receptors. It does not appear to deplete dopamine stores.

E FALSE Lithium is used to treat psychoses, but it is thought to act by entering cells together with Na^+ to create an intracellular surplus of cations and so decrease the resting membrane potential.

Central Nervous System — General: related questions 2, 17, 26, 140, 192

162 Anxiolytic drugs

    A are major tranquillisers
    B are hypnotics
    C are sedatives
    D produce a harmful interaction with alcohol
    E produce a harmful interaction with aspirin

A FALSE The major tranquilliser group of drugs (e.g. chlorpromazine, haloperidol) are antipsychotic agents used in the treatment of mania and schizophrenia. The anxiolytic agents are used to treat anxiety neuroses and include the benzodiazepines, barbiturates, and propanediols.

B TRUE All anxiolytic drugs when administered at higher doses become sedative, and at even higher doses are hypnotic. They depress electrical activity in the thalamus, reticular activating system and the cortex, actions which one would expect progressively to lower mental tension and anxiety, to cause apathy and eventually to induce drowsiness and sleep.

C TRUE See B.

D TRUE As a general rule central depressant drugs have their action potentiated by ethyl alcohol and anxiolytic drugs are no exception.

E FALSE Aspirin produces interactions with many drugs, some of which may prove fatal. They are generally related to the ability of aspirin to displace drugs from circulating plasma protein. No important interactions have been reported with anxiolytic drugs.

163 Benzodiazepines

    A unlike barbiturates do not produce tolerance or physical dependence

    B powerfully induce hepatic enzyme systems

    C do not effect sleeping electroencephalogram (eeg) patterns

    D have so little respiratory depressant effect that they may safely be used in patients with obstructive airways disease

    E are sometimes used to relax spastic muscles

A FALSE Habituation with benzodiazepines is common, but tolerance and physical dependence can also occur following chronic administration. The withdrawal syndrome is usually benign, except after large doses when convulsions may occur. The withdrawal response may be delayed by up to a week because of the long half-life of these drugs.

B FALSE Although metabolised by the liver, these drugs do not significantly induce microsomal enzymes and apart from additive effects with other cns depressants, interactions are rare.

C FALSE Sleep is accompanied by characteristic changes in the eeg pattern which alter in a cyclical manner throughout the night. During orthodox sleep there are large slow eeg waves with runs of fast activity called 'sleep spindles'; during paradoxical sleep the eeg shows runs of low voltage slow waves. Bursts of rapid-eye-movement (rem) occur during this stage, and are preceded by a run of sharp waves on the eeg. All hypnotics produce sleep in which the total amount of rem sleep and the accompanying eeg changes are reduced, although benzodiazepines seem to cause less reduction than the barbiturates. The rebound increase in rem sleep (in which vivid and frightening dreams may occur) that follows withdrawal of hypnotics is also less severe with the benzodiazepines.

D FALSE The therapeutic ratio of the benzodiazepines is very high, and it is generally agreed that in subjects with normal respiratory function, these drugs have negligible effect. Nevertheless, there is good evidence that in patients with broncho-pulmonary disease, depression of respiration occurs, possibly due to carbon dioxide narcosis.

E TRUE The acute muscle spasm which may follow trauma and inflammation may be relieved by benzodiazepines (in particular diazepam). The muscle relaxation is primarily due to an action of the drugs on reticular neuronal mechanisms controlling muscle tone, but a spinal site may also be involved.

164 Barbiturates

A can cause confusion in the elderly

B other than phenobarbitone are excreted primarily unchanged in the urine

C may interfere with oral anticoagulant therapy

D when taken in overdose cause sedation which should be treated with stimulant drugs

E all possess anticonvulsant activity

A TRUE Excitement and confusion are common features seen in elderly patients when barbiturates are prescribed as hypnotics. It is less likely to occur with the benzodiazepines.

B FALSE Only phenobarbitone (about 50 per cent) and barbitone (about 8 per cent) are excreted unchanged in the urine to any significant extent. The barbiturates commonly used as hypnotics or sedatives, like pentobarbitone, and intravenous anaesthetics, like thiopentone, are first metabolised in the liver.

C TRUE By inducing liver microsomal enzyme systems, the chronic use of barbiturates will interfere with the action of other drugs; and oral anticoagulants, like warfarin, which are normally metabolised by this enzyme system will have a shorter and less profound action than expected.

D FALSE Stimulant (analeptic) drugs have no part in the treatment of barbiturate overdose. Sometimes, it is possible to prevent sedation by lowering the dose, as in the treatment of epilepsy, but if sedation is due to acute overdose with a medium/short acting barbiturate then other measures are necessary, i.e. maintenance of respiration, blood pressure and body temperature. Forced diuresis or haemodialysis are only of value with phenobarbitone and barbitone (see B). Removal of other barbiturates from the blood, where supportive measures have failed, would require charcoal or resin haemoperfusion.

E FALSE Barbiturates have the following general structure, and variation in the substituent groups produces a wide range of pharmacological activity.

$$
\begin{array}{c}
R_3 \\
\backslash \\
N \text{---} C \quad R_1 \\
/ \qquad \backslash \ / \\
X \text{==} C \qquad C \\
\backslash \qquad / \ \backslash \\
N \text{---} C \quad R_2 \\
/ \qquad \parallel \\
H \qquad O
\end{array}
$$

A phenyl group at R_3 or R_2 confers selective anticonvulsant activity as in phenobarbitone, but if a long alkyl group is substituted at either of these sites, hypnotic activity will diminish and convulsant properties may appear.

165 Which of the following is/are metabolised more rapidly in patients chronically exposed to barbiturates

A cholecalciferol
B ethinyl oestradiol
C digoxin
D penicillin G
E streptomycin

Note: Chronic administration of barbiturates causes increased production of the non-specific microsomal enzymes in the liver a process commonly referred to as 'enzyme induction'. This has the effect of increasing the metabolism not only of the barbiturate but also of a number of other drugs and hormones.

A TRUE Cholecalciferol (vitamin D_3) is available in the body either from the diet or by conversion of 7-dehydrocholesterol in the skin following exposure to ultraviolet irradiation. To perform its physiological role in calcium metabolism cholecalciferol must undergo metabolic activation, and the first step in this process is brought about by liver microsomal enzymes. It is thought that barbiturates may interfere at this stage by inducing inactivating enzymes and as a result cause osteomalacia (i.e. defective mineralisation of bone).

B TRUE Ethinyl oestradiol is widely used as the oestrogenic component of the combined oral contraceptive pill. It is normally only slowly metabolised by the liver (a fact which explains is much greater potency than the endogenous oestrogens), but in women in whom liver microsomal enzymes have been induced, its action is reduced and breakthrough bleeding may occur.

C FALSE Elimination of digoxin in man is mainly by renal excretion, some 60 to 90 per cent being excreted unchanged in the urine. It is removed by glomerular filtration, and sensitivity to digoxin increases in old age as the filtration rate declines. Less than 10 per cent is metabolised by the liver, and neither hepatic disease nor chronic barbiturate administration significantly alter its efficacy.

D FALSE Following injection, between 60 to 90 per cent of penicillin G is removed from the circulation by the kidney, mostly by tubular secretion, and unless given in a form in which absorption is delayed, it has a half-life in the body of only half an hour. The remainder is excreted in the bile, but barbiturate administration does not significantly affect its metabolism.

E FALSE Streptomycin is excreted primarily by glomerular filtration, and whilst impaired renal function will noticeably increase toxicity (especially ototoxicity) change in hepatic function of the type produced by barbiturates does not alter its action.

166 Nitrazepam is considered a useful hypnotic because normal therapy does not produce significant

    A addiction
    B respiratory depression
    C hangover
    D increased cns depression with ethyl alcohol
    E rebound dreaming on withdrawal

A FALSE Tolerance and physical dependence do occur following chronic use of nitrazepam but unless large doses are given the withdrawal syndrome is relatively mild. With large doses convulsions may follow withdrawal, but because of the long half-life of the drug they may not occur until several days after the last dose.

B TRUE Nitrazepam like other benzodiazepines has a high therapeutic ratio and it is generally agreed that in subjects with normal respiratory function there is no respiratory depression unless many times the therapeutic dose is given.

C FALSE Benzodiazepines have gained the reputation of producing only a mild hangover and many patients experience no subjective after effects. However, objective studies have shown both mental acuity and reaction time to be depressed for many hours after waking and to be similar to the action of amylobarbitone.

D FALSE Alcohol increases the cns depressant actions produced by all centrally acting drugs, and nitrazepam is no exception. In fact, of the deaths attributed to nitrazepam, many have involved consumption of alcohol as well.

E FALSE Nitrazepam produces some suppression of rem sleep but it is much less than with barbiturates. Nevertheless, it is sufficient to induce a rebound increase of rem (dream) sleep on withdrawal, and to produce other features of withdrawal such as irritability and perhaps even insomnia.

167 Chloral hydrate

    A is a respiratory depressant
    B may cause gastritis
    C is metabolised to trichloroethanol which is an effective hypnotic
    D can cause tolerance and drug dependence
    E toxicity is much increased by simultaneous administration of ethanol

---

A TRUE Like other hypnotic agents, chloral hydrate produces a general and progressive depression of the cns, and although at normal doses respiratory depression is not apparent, large doses depress both the respiratory and cardiovascular systems, and even normal doses can precipitate respiratory failure in patients with chronic respiratory disease.

B TRUE Chloral hydrate is irritating to the skin and mucous membranes, and if taken on an empty stomach or if insufficiently diluted may cause gastritis. The phosphate ester of chloral hydrate, namely triclofos which is given in tablet form, releases only a little chloral into the stomach and is virtually non-irritant. It also lacks the disagreeable taste of chloral hydrate.

C TRUE Chloral hydrate is reduced to trichloroethanol in the liver and kidney as follows:

$$\underset{\substack{| \\ Cl}}{\overset{\substack{Cl\quad H}}{Cl - C - C - OH}}\,\underset{OH}{\overset{H}{}} + NADPH + H^+ \xrightarrow[\text{dehydrogenase}]{\text{alcohol}} \underset{\substack{| \quad | \\ Cl \quad H}}{\overset{\substack{Cl\quad H}}{Cl - C - C - OH}} + NADP^+ + H_2O$$

Both chloral hydrate and trichloroethanol are hypnotic, but the latter, because it is less polar, and because following metabolism it quickly becomes the major component, is responsible for most of the central action.

D TRUE Following the habitual use of chloral hydrate both tolerance and physical dependence occur. This form of addiction is similar to alcoholism and withdrawal may result in delirium. Gastritis and skin eruptions are common features.

E TRUE Ethyl alcohol laced with chloral hydrate is the traditional knockout mixture known as a 'Mickey Finn'; and although some experiments have indicated that this mixture may not be as potent as is generally believed, a combination of two central depressants produces at least an additive effect on the cns, and where one of the agents is alcohol, the depression may be supra-additive.

Central Nervous System — Anxiolytics, sedatives and hypnotics: related questions 24, 27, 28

168 When receiving monoamine oxidase inhibitors (MAOIs) for the treatment of depression

    A maprotyline will have a potentiated action
    B paracetamol should not be administered
    C local anaesthetics containing felypressin should not be used
    D cold remedies containing nasal decongestants should not be used
    E ingestion of yeast extracts may provoke a hypotensive crisis

---

A TRUE Maprotyline is a newer antidepressant which like the tricyclics inhibits the re-uptake of noradrenaline into neurones within the cns. MAOIs produce a similar antidepressant effect by preventing the breakdown of noradrenaline so that the amounts released following nerve stimulation are much greater.

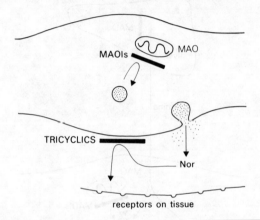

When used together a much increased effect is seen and such combination therapy has been used to treat depression, but toxic interactions may occur.

B FALSE Although paracetamol is metabolised by the liver and MAOIs do inhibit microsomal enzyme systems at this site, the action of paracetamol does not appear to be modified by such treatment.

C FALSE Felypressin is a polypeptide vasoconstrictor agent added to the local anaesthetic prilocaine to potentiate and prolong its local action. There is no evidence that its action is modified by treatment with MAOIs.

D TRUE The nasal decongestants commonly added to proprietary cold preparations include ephedrine, phenylephrine and phenylpropranolamine. At least part of the action of such compounds is to release noradrenaline from sympathetic neurones and, since following treatment with MAOIs the neurones contain larger than normal stores of noradrenaline, these indirectly acting amines release correspondingly greater amounts. A hypertensive crisis may follow such an interaction.

E FALSE Yeast extracts contain large amounts of tyramine which is an indirectly acting amine (see D). The tyramine is normally destroyed by MAO in the gastrointestinal tract and liver and does not have a pharmacological action. In the presence of MAOIs the tyramine releases noradrenaline from the neuronal stores to cause massive vasoconstriction and a potential dangerous *hypertension*.

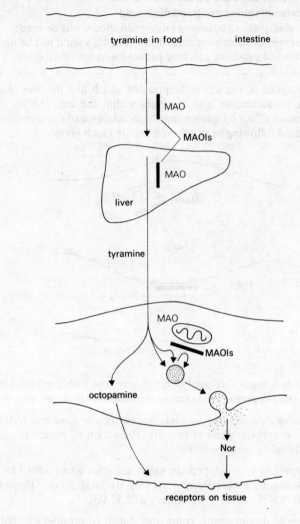

169 Cheese should not be allowed in the diet of patients being given monoamine oxidase inhibitors (MAOIs) because

    A mental depression can result
    B the blood pressure will be elevated
    C cheese contains tyrosine
    D it interferes with the metabolism of the MAOIs
    E substances are present in cheese that cause release of noradrenaline from stores in the body

---

A FALSE MAOIs are used in the clinical treatment of depression and although they interfere with the metabolism of a number of drugs and foods, which as a consequence produce untoward effects, such substances do not apparently modify the antidepressant effect of the MAOIs.

B TRUE As a result of the action of tyramine (see C), massive peripheral vaso-constriction occurs. This elevates the blood pressure sufficiently, at the very least to produce an unpleasant headache, but in extreme cases to cause intracranial bleeding and perhaps death. Such hypertensive crises can be treated by giving a short acting α-blocker, e.g. phentolamine.

C FALSE Tyrosine is an amino acid and is undoubtedly present in cheese. When absorbed it is without pharmacological effect and the use of MAOIs does not appear to modify this. Cheese also contains tyramine which is normally inactivated by MAO in the gut and liver. When the activity of the enzyme has been inhibited the tyramine can enter the general circulation to produce release of noradrenaline from sympathetic nerves throughout the body (see E). The result of this is described in B.

D FALSE There is no evidence that consumption of cheese in any way alters the metabolism of MAOIs even though these compounds differ widely in their structures and therefore in their route of inactivation.

E TRUE Tyramine present in cheese is an indirectly acting sympathomimetic amine. In the presence of MAOIs it is not inactivated and enters the circulation to be taken up into sympathetic nerves by the Uptake I process to bring about release of noradrenaline from storage sites. Larger than normal stores of amine are present in the nerve due to the inhibition of intraneuronal MAO, so that marked sympathomimetic effects are produced (see B). Tyramine is also converted to octopamine which is released, along with noradrenaline, to produce a direct effect on the receptors.

170 A potentially harmful interaction may occur if a patient taking tricyclic anti-depressants also receives

    A milk

    B cheese

    C a monoamine oxidase inhibitor (MAOI)

    D local anaesthetics containing adrenaline

    E paracetamol

Note: The tricyclic antidepressants do not interfere significantly with the metabolism of other drugs; the most important interactions are pharmacodynamic ones due to modification of the pharmacological effect of other agents.

A FALSE Milk does not normally interfere with the action of drugs except in some circumstances to delay absorption. Exceptions to this rule are the tetra-cyclines which form insoluble chelates with the Ca^{++} in milk.

B FALSE Cheese is contraindicated when using monoamine oxidase inhibitor antidepressants because the tyramine that it contains is not metabolised, and a dangerous hypertension may result. The tricyclics do not suffer from this dis-advantage (see Note).

C TRUE Tricyclic antidepressants prevent the re-uptake of noradrenaline into the nerve (Uptake 1) after passage of the nerve impulse. MAOIs, by preventing intraneuronal metabolism of noradrenaline, increase the vesicular stores and thus the amount of amine that is released following nerve stimulation. When used together the actions of the drugs become additive, and dangerous hypertension, excitement and hyperpyrexia may occur. Nevertheless, by reducing the dose of each drug, it is possible to use them together and many psychiatrists claim that the combination is effective in patients where either group alone has failed.

D TRUE When injected into the circulation, adrenaline is inactivated largely by uptake into neuronal stores (Uptake 1). Because the tricyclic antidepressants block this process, the actions of adrenaline will be prolonged and potentiated. With local anaesthetics containing adrenaline, this is only likely to be of importance if the drug is inadvertently injected into a blood vessel, when potentially harmful arrhyth-mias might occur. In practice, the risk is small, but it is wise not to take it.

E FALSE No interactions between these two drugs have been reported, nor, from what is known of their mechanisms of action and inactivation, would any be anticipated.

171 Caffeine

A antagonises fatigue
B increases intracellular cyclic AMP (cAMP) levels
C is diuretic
D enhances cns reflex activity
E in large doses increases myocardial excitability

A TRUE Caffeine is well known as a cns stimulant, affecting progressively all parts of the brain. The cortex is first to experience the action, followed by the medulla and then the spinal cord. The actions on the cortex include clearer thought, reduced drowsiness and fatigue, and increased ability to maintain intellectual effort.

B TRUE Caffeine increases intracellular levels of cAMP by inhibiting its breakdown by phosphodiesterase. The resulting effects on the heart, lungs, vasculature and cns are thus similar to those seen with sympathomimetic agents.

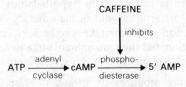

C TRUE Methylxanthines like caffeine are diuretics. At least part of their action is due to the increased renal blood flow and glomerular filtration rate that follow cardiac stimulation. However, they also have a direct action on the renal tubules to increase Na^+ and Cl^- excretion. The overal diuresis is small, and caffeine is not useful clinically for this purpose.

D TRUE Following the cortical action (see A) of relatively small amounts of caffeine (1 to 2 cups of coffee or tea), conditioned reflexes are enhanced. Thus, the reaction times to visual and auditory stimuli are reduced, and the rate of performing repetitive motor tasks (e.g. typing) is increased. At larger doses, caffeine stimulates progressively the whole cns. At a spinal level, the effect is to increase reflex excitability, and to stimulate lower motor centres. In experimental animals, this may lead to clonic convulsions, but such an effect in man is virtually unknown.

E TRUE The effect of increasing intracellular cAMP levels (see B) in the myocardium is to produce both positive inotropic and chronotropic actions. Palpitations, and even extrasystoles have been reported in subjects who consume large amounts of strong coffee.

172 Amphetamine

A reduces hyperactivity in children
B increases appetite
C is a selective β-adrenergic agonist
D l-isomer has greater cns stimulant activity than the d-isomer
E increases restlessness

A TRUE Amphetamine has a dramatic effect in calming some abnormally hyper-active children. The restlessness, ease of distraction and impulsive behaviour associated with the condition are reduced, and the child becomes more attentive, calmer and altogether more co-operative. Whilst the increased alertness and greater concentration are explicable in terms of the central actions of amphetamine, the calming action appears paradoxical.

B FALSE Amphetamine reduces appetite, the site of action being most probably the so-called feeding centre in the lateral hypothalamus. In animals the effect is marked and may lead to starvation, but in man dietary control is an essential adjunct if adequate reduction of food intake is to be achieved. Because of the powerful psychological addiction and the schizophrenia-like psychosis that chronic use of this drug can cause, amphetamine is no longer widely used in clinical medicine.

C FALSE Amphetamine produces its stimulant effects in two ways: first, by causing release of catecholamines from adrenergic neurones and secondly, by preventing re-uptake of such amines back into the nerve (i.e. inhibition of Uptake I). The result is that both α and β actions become apparent.

D FALSE Amphetamine (3-phenylisopropylamine) is a racemic mixture of which the d-rotatory isomer (dexamphetamine) has the more potent action (about 4 times that of the l-isomer).

E TRUE The potent stimulant effects of amphetamine on the cns include elevated mood, increased confidence, delayed fatigue and increased motor and speech activity. However, in many individuals (and certainly following overdose) headache palpitations, restlessness, agitation, apprehension and confusion may accompany its use.

Central Nervous System — Stimulants and antidepressants: related questions 22, 23, 24

173 Which of the following drugs are useful in calming severely disturbed and aggressive patients

    A amitryptiline
    B haloperidol
    C chlorpromazine
    D tranylcypromine
    E phenytoin

A FALSE Amitryptiline is one of the most widely used tricyclic antidepressant drugs. It is mildly tranquillising and may cause drowsiness and is of particular value in depressed patients who are agitated and who have disturbed sleep. Despite this, the general action of the drug is mood elevating which would not be appropriate treatment for disturbed or aggressive patients.

B TRUE Chemically, haloperidol is a butyrophenone, and like chlorpromazine, it is a receptor antagonist of dopamine in the cns. It is powerful (weight for weight more potent than chlorpromazine) and especially useful in manic psychoses. The blockade of dopamine receptors leads to dose related extrapyramidal side effects, but loss of appetite, depressive reactions and occasionally liver damage are also seen.

C TRUE Classified as a major tranquilliser, chlorpromazine has a well established role in the treatment of mania and schizophrenia. It is thought to work primarily through its ability to block dopamine receptors. Extrapyramidal symptoms may complicate its use.

D FALSE Related in structure to amphetamine, the monoamine oxidase inhibitor tranylcypromine also has direct sympathomimetic actions. It is one of the safest and most widely used of this class of drugs. It is used in the treatment of depression.

E FALSE Phenytoin is an anticonvulsant used in the treatment of grand mal epilepsy, and although in high doses it produces sedation, it is not a useful drug for treating disturbed and aggressive patients.

174 Which of the following is/are true of chlorpromazine
  A it is antipsychotic because of its ability to stimulate dopamine receptors
  B it is an α-adrenoceptor blocker
  C its antiemetic activity is due to blockade of the vagus
  D hypothermia is produced because of hypothalamic inhibition
  E hepatocellular jaundice may occur

A FALSE Chlorpromazine blocks dopamine receptors, and whilst the detailed mechanism by which drugs produce their antipsychotic action is still far from clear, there is much evidence to suggest that a major part of their action is due to dopamine antagonism. Part of this evidence is that all the major tranquillisers cause extrapyramidal effects (i.e. Parkinsonism) which is known to be due to dopamine insufficiency, and drugs which deplete central amine stores (e.g. reserpine) are antipsychotic in action.

B TRUE Chlorpromazine is an α-blocking drug and has been used to overcome the sympathetic vasoconstriction that occurs during cardiogenic shock.

C FALSE Like other phenothiazines, chlorpromazine is a powerful antiemetic, but its action is not on the vagus, it is on the chemoreceptor trigger zone (ctz) in the area postrema of the medulla. The effect occurs at lower doses than the antipsychotic action and since it blocks the emetic effect of the dopamine receptor stimulant, apomorphine, it would appear to act by blocking dopamine receptors. It will not control vomiting of vestibular origin, e.g. motion sickness (see diagram Q140, page 161).

D TRUE By inhibiting the action of dopaminergic neurones in the hypothalamus, chlorpromazine lowers body temperature and reduces release of pituitary hormones. In fact, chlorpromazine was introduced into clinical medicine as an agent that induced a tranquil condition and a lowered body temperature, properties that potentiated the action of general anaesthetics and produced a condition described as 'artificial hibernation'.

E FALSE Between 1 to 4 per cent of patients receiving chlorpromazine develop a type of jaundice described as hepatic cholestasis in which there is stasis of bile in the liver cells and canaliculi, as if there was an obstruction in the bile duct. An increase in the viscosity of the bile seems to be the cause. Hepatocellular jaundice refers to the condition associated with viral hepatitis and cirrhosis in which there is diffuse liver cell injury, causing impaired uptake, conjugations and excretion by the liver.

175 Common toxic effects of chlorpromazine include
A dystonic reaction
B hallucinations
C elation
D anxiety
E extrapyramidal effects

A TRUE When therapy with chlorpromazine is initiated an acute dystonic reaction may occur, the features of which include facial grimacing, torticollis (involuntary movements of neck muscles) and oculogyric crises. It is an extrapyramidal effect of the drug (see E) and unlike hysterical reactions, for which they may be mistaken, it responds to antiparkinsonian drugs.

B FALSE Hallucinations are a common feature of psychoses and are generally controlled by the use of chlorpromazine.

C FALSE Chlorpromazine is a major tranquilliser used to control the mania and disturbed moods of psychotic patients. As the classification suggests, its overall action is to induce a tranquil state and to control the abnormal elation seen in psychotic patients. Excessive action may lead to depression.

D FALSE On the whole, the action of major tranquillisers is to induce a diminished emotional response to external stimuli, and chlorpromazine will, therefore, control the psychotic agitation and hyperactivity which are a feature of schizophrenia. Such drugs are not, however, used to treat anxiety neuroses.

E TRUE Because of its ability to block dopamine, chlorpromazine induces a number of neurological side effects due to an action in the extrapyramidal system. The syndromes are as follows:

1. Parkinsonism − indistinguishable from idiopathic disease.
2. Akathisia − where the patient has a compulsion to keep moving.
3. Dystonic reactions − see A.
4. Tardive dyskinesia − occurs much later than the other effects, and is characterised by stereotyped jaw and tongue movements, lip smacking and sucking.

176 Lithium

    A can terminate an attack of mania
    B can prevent an attack of mania
    C causes tremor
    D may produce a goitre
    E produces megaloblastic anaemia

A TRUE Given as the carbonate, lithium in normal man has no discernible psychotropic action, and unlike the phenothiazines, is not sedative. However, in patients, lithium has proved a useful agent to treat both mania and hypomania. It is used as a maintenance therapy, and as a primary treatment of acute episodes.

B TRUE See A.

C TRUE Fatigue, muscle weakness, slurred speech, ataxia and a fine tremor are motor dysfunctions commonly seen following treatment with lithium. Whilst many of the side effects disappear after a week or so, the tremor persists.

D TRUE Lithium has an action on the thyroid gland similar to that produced by iodide, and there is evidence of impaired thyroid hormone secretion in most patients treated with the drug. In a small proportion of patients the impaired uptake of iodide is sufficient to induce hyperstimulation of the gland cells and cause goitre.

E FALSE An increase in circulating leukocytes occurs during lithium treatment, but megaloblastic anaemia is not a feature of toxicity.

177 In the treatment of Parkinson's disease

   A benzhexol stimulates cholinergic receptors
   B amantadine blocks cholinergic receptors
   C reserpine is effective because it depletes stores of amines from neurones throughout the cns
   D chlorpromazine is contraindicated
   E decarboxylase inhibitors like carbidopa (α-methyl dopa hydrazine) are useful because they have a selective action on the cns

Note: Normal control of the extrapyramidal system is maintained by a balance between acetyl-choline (an excitatory transmitter) and dopamine (an inhibitory transmitter) acting on cell bodies in the corpus striatum. In Parkinsonism, where dopamine levels are deficient, the acetyl-choline produces greater than normal effect and impairment of the quality and smoothness of voluntary movement results.

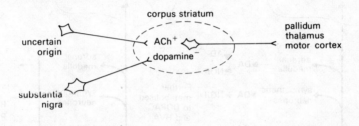

A FALSE Benzhexol is a muscarinic blocker and is effective because it reduces the cholinergic dominance (see Note). It controls the rigidity of the disease but not the tremor, and its use is accompanied, as one might expect, by anticholinergic problems, i.e. dry mouth, blurred vision, etc.

B FALSE Amantadine is strictly an antiviral agent, but is also of value in Parkinsonism, primarily because it stimulates release of dopamine from neurones in the striatum. It also has some stimulant effect directly on the dopamine receptors, but it only produces a useful action when the dopaminergic neurones in the nigro-striatal pathway are still functioning.

C FALSE By blocking incorporation of amines into vesicles in both central and peripheral aminergic neurones, reserpine depletes the nerves of transmitter and causes failure of transmission. Noradrenaline, adrenaline, dopamine and 5-hydroxy-tryptamine (5-HT) containing neurones are affected, and the action in Parkinsonism would be to deplete still further the deficient dopaminergic neurones in the nigro-striatal pathway. Such an action would make the condition worse.

D TRUE The major tranquilliser, chlorpromazine, can antagonise the action of many central transmitters (e.g. acetylcholine, noradrenaline, adrenaline, 5-HT, dopamine and histamine). Even in patients without signs of existing extrapyramidal disturbance, the impairment of dopamine action may lead to Parkinsonian symptoms, but in patients already demonstrating this disease, the condition will be exacerbated. Chlorpromazine is contraindicated in such patients.

E FALSE Dopamine cannot be given to treat Parkinsonism because it does not pass the blood/brain barrier in significant amounts. Instead, levodopa is administered which must first be converted in vivo to dopamine. Such metabolism is brought about by the enzyme dopa decarboxylase, but herein lies a snag in that considerable peripheral conversion of levodopa occurs. This leads to diminished central action and the appearance of peripheral toxicity. Carbidopa inhibits dopa decarboxylase but it does not cross the blood/brain barrier, so that peripheral conversion of levodopa falls, peripheral side effects are less, and the dose of levodopa can be reduced.

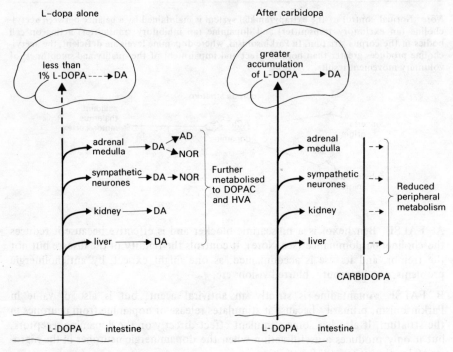

DOPAC = dihydroxyphenylacetic acid
HVA = homovanillic acid

178 Levodopa diminishes the symptoms of Parkinsonism because
   A   it is converted to dopamine in the cns
   B   there is a deficiency of dopamine in the brains of patients with this
       disease
   C   it blocks cholinergic receptors in the corpus striatum
   D   it is converted to noradrenaline in sympathetic neurones
   E   it is an inhibitory transmitter

A   TRUE   Parkinsonism is associated with a deficiency of dopamine in the extra-pyramidal system of the brain (see B). This deficiency can be rectified by giving levodopa, which is readily metabolised by dopa decarboxylase in the central neurones to dopamine. Treatment with levodopa alleviates mainly the akinesia and rigidity but has less effect on the tremor.

B   TRUE   Normal control of the extrapyramidal system is maintained by a balance between acetylcholine (an excitatory transmitter) and dopamine (an inhibitory transmitter) acting on cell bodies in the corpus striatum. In Parkinsonism there is a deficiency of dopamine so that the acetylcholine produces a greater than normal effect. This impairs the quality and smoothness of voluntary movement.

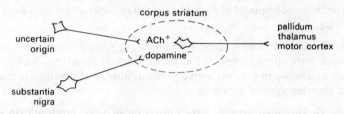

C   FALSE   Although it is possible to alleviate some aspects of Parkinsonism by administering muscarinic blockers (e.g. benzhexol), cholinergic blockade is not an action of either dopa or dopamine.

D   FALSE   Less than 1 per cent of an administered dose of levodopa enters the cns to be converted to dopamine in the extrapyramidal system. The vast majority of the remaining dopa is converted to dopamine by aromatic-l-amino acid decarboxylase, primarily in the liver, but also in sympathetic neurones and the adrenal medulla. A small proportion of such dopamine will be converted to noradrenaline, but biotransformation is mainly to dihydroxyphenylacetic acid (DOPAC) and homovanillic acid (HVA). Conversion of dopa to noradrenaline outside the cns is not thought to be essential to the treatment of Parkinsonism; on the contrary, if peripheral metabolism of levodopa is inhibited (e.g. with carbidopa) larger amounts enter the cns and therapy becomes more effective.

E   FALSE   It is dopamine (not levodopa) that is the inhibitory transmitter (see B).

179 Treatment of Parkinsonism with levodopa may

    A reduce nausea and vomiting
    B relieve rigidity
    C improve depression
    D induce mental illness
    E cause hypertension

A FALSE Nausea and vomiting is not characteristic of Parkinsonism, but is a common feature following treatment of patients with levodopa. It occurs mainly when the dose is being increased, and can be reduced to a minimum by increasing the dose slowly and taking the drug after food to delay absorption.

B TRUE Rigidity is one of the three main symptoms of Parkinsonism (the other two are tremor and akinesia). In the early stages of the disease, it is manifested as severe cramp, but then becomes a resistance of the limb to passive movement. If the resistance is constant, it is described as 'lead pipe', if it is intermittent as 'cogwheel'. Levodopa generally alleviates the rigidity and the akinesia, but produces less improvement of the tremor.

C TRUE A common symptom of Parkinsonism is depression, and following treatment with levodopa mild elation in mood may occur which may even progress to hypomania.

D TRUE Paranoid delusions, depressive illness, aggression, suicidal behaviour and hallucinations have all been reported in patients taking levodopa. Such effects are more likely to develop in patients with a previous history of psychiatric disturbance or in those showing signs of dementia.

E FALSE Parkinsonian patients have a lower mean blood pressure than would be expected for their age, and following treatment with levodopa this will be lowered still further. About one third of patients develop significant orthostatic hypotension which in a few patients will be accompanied by dizziness and even fainting. Fortunately tolerance to this effect develops as treatment progresses.

180 Parkinsonism may be aggravated by

A promethazine
B haloperidol
C anticholinesterase drugs
D diazepam
E bromocriptine

A FALSE Although promethazine is a phenothiazine, unlike the related substance chlorpromazine it does not possess antipsychotic activity, and does not antagonise the action of dopamine; and whereas chlorpromazine will induce Parkinsonism, promethazine is without effect. In fact, some degree of improvement may occur due to the anticholinergic activity of this drug.

B TRUE Haloperidol is a butyrophenone with powerful antipsychotic activity. It is a receptor antagonist of dopamine in the cns, and as such will reduce the efficacy of the already depleted output of dopamine from the nigrostriatal neurones in Parkinsonian patients. Its use in this disease is contraindicated.

C TRUE In Parkinsonism the reduced output of the inhibitory transmitter dopamine means that excitatory cholinergic activity goes unchecked (see diagram Q177, page 201). Administration of an anticholinesterase drug would, if it penetrated into the cns, make matters worse.

D FALSE There is no evidence that diazepam exacerbates Parkinsonism. On the contrary, since the condition may well be aggravated by anxiety, treatment with these drugs may actually be beneficial.

E FALSE Bromocriptine is a stimulant of dopaminergic receptors, and as such has been used to overcome the dopamine deficiency of Parkinsonism and to treat some forms of infertility where it causes inhibition of prolactin secretion.

181 Which of the following give effective treatment of petit mal

   A ethosuximide
   B carbamazepine
   C primidone
   D sodium valproate
   E clonazepam

Note: Petit mal refers to the epileptic condition in which the patient commonly has brief periods (10 to 15 seconds) of unconsciousness. Such 'absences' may occur many times a day and may be accompanied by myoclonic jerks of the arms. Bilateral synchronous spike and slow wave complexes with a frequency of 3 cycle/sec accompany the attacks.

A TRUE Ethosuximide is one of a series of succinimide derivatives which is effective orally in the treatment of petit mal. The dose must be adjusted to the patient to maintain an effective blood concentration without toxicity. It is of no value in grand mal, but may be used in conjunction with anticonvulsants where petit mal and other forms of epilepsy coexist.

B FALSE Carbamazepine is used in the treatment of grand mal and psycho-motor epilepsy and is probably most useful in adults. It does not, however, provide adequate control of 'absences'. It is also effective in treating trigeminal neuralgia.

C FALSE Closely related to phenobarbitone, and partly converted to it by liver enzymes, primidone is also a sedative anticonvulsant. It has a similar range of usefulness namely grand mal and psychomotor epilepsy.

D TRUE This anticonvulsant is unusual in that the chemical structure contains no nitrogen atom and because it inhibits the metabolism of gamma-amino-butyric acid (GABA) (an action that may account for its antiepileptic effects). It will control infantile spasms, myoclonic epilepsies and is the drug of choice in patients with absences and 3 cycle/sec spike and wave discharges in the eeg.

E TRUE As the name suggests, clonazepam is a benzodiazepine and is probably the most effective anticonvulsant in the series. They all suppress the spontaneous eeg changes in petit mal seizures, and are effective intravenously in the control of status epilepticus. Long term oral use is complicated by sedation and the development of tolerance.

182 In the treatment of grand mal epilepsy

  A carbamazepine is effective

  B phenytoin is particularly useful because plasma levels correlate well with the dose of the drug

  C clonazepam is effective

  D in children, sodium valproate should *not* be prescribed

  E primidone does *not* cause sedation

A TRUE Carbamazepine is an anticonvulsant drug used in the treatment of both grand mal and psychomotor epilepsy, often in conjunction with other drugs. Frequent blood counts and tests of liver function during its use may help to avoid toxicity. It is often preferred to the barbiturates because it causes less sedation.

B FALSE Blood levels reflect very well the state of the patient and the efficacy of the drug. Thus, optimal control of fits is normally obtained at blood levels of 10 to 20 μg/ml, ataxia develops by 30 μg/ml, and over 40 μg/ml the patient will demonstrate lethargy and sedation. Unfortunately, because of wide individual variation in the rate of metabolism, blood levels cannot be accurately predicted from the administered daily dose of drug in any given patient, and in order to ensure adequate therapy without toxicity, measurement of blood levels may be necessary.

C TRUE Clonazepam is a benzodiazepine which may be used in the treatment of all types of epilepsy and seizure. In grand mal epilepsy, it is mainly used to supplement other forms of treatment, where control of the disease is inadequate.

D FALSE Sodium valproate is regarded by many as the best drug for the treatment of children, partly because it has remarkably little toxicity (occasional nausea and vomiting) and partly because the alternatives are limited by toxicity. Phenobarbitone and primidone, for example, may produce behavioural disturbances; and phenytoin readily causes drowsiness and lethargy which retards learning.

E FALSE Chemically related to phenobarbitone, and partly converted to it by liver enzymes, primidone produces similar toxicity to phenobarbitone. This includes sedation and cerebellar ataxia. Some patients are intolerant to primidone and a small test dose is recommended.

183 Phenytoin

    A is metabolised by zero order kinetics
    B is effective in petit mal
    C is effective in psychomotor epilepsy
    D inhibits hepatic enzyme systems
    E produces sedation at anticonvulsant plasma levels

A TRUE At plasma concentrations below about 10 μg/ml, phenytoin metabolism is exponential. In other words as substrate concentration rises so does the rate of elimination, and the half-life regardless of dose remains constant (on average about 2 hours). This is described as first order kinetics. At higher concentrations, the enzyme system becomes saturated or is inhibited by metabolites and the half-life increases, i.e. zero order kinetics apply.

B FALSE Phenytoin, in common with phenobarbitone and primidone, is not effective against petit mal, and may actually increase the frequency of attacks.

C TRUE Temporal lobe or psychomotor epilepsy, which is characterised by attacks of confused behaviour not always accompanied by major convulsions, accounts for about one third of all cases of epilepsy. It is more refractory to treatment than grand mal; phenytoin and primidone are the drugs of choice.

D FALSE Phenytoin is metabolised primarily by hepatic microsomal enzymes. The majority is hydroxylated and although high levels of the drug readily saturate the enzyme, inhibition does not occur; in fact chronic use may lead to mild enzyme induction and therefore more rapid metabolism.

E FALSE Optimal control of fits is usually obtained with blood concentrations in the range of 10 to 20 μg/ml, although levels below this may be effective in some patients. Nystagmus is usually apparent by 20 μg/ml, ataxia by 30 μg/ml, but lethargy and sedation do not normally occur until the blood level exceeds 40 μg/ml. The main problem in treatment is the variable relationship between daily dose and blood concentration in individual patients, and assessment of blood levels may be necessary to establish the correct regime for a given subject.

184 Phenytoin toxicity includes

    A cardiac dysrhythmia
    B Parkinsonian tremors
    C loss of hair
    D cerebellar dysfunction
    E gingival hypertrophy

A FALSE The membrane stabilising activity of phenytoin that makes it useful in controlling excessive electrical activity in the brain also makes it of value in treating cardiac dysrhythmias. Its action is similar to that of lignocaine but it has been found to be especially useful in the treatment of digitalis-induced ventricular dysrhythmias.

B FALSE Hyperactivity, silliness, confusion, ataxia and hyperactive tendon reflexes are some of the toxic actions of phenytoin on the cns, but extrapyramidal effects likely to cause Parkinsonian tremors are not seen.

C FALSE On the contrary, hirsutism is a common manifestation, being particularly disturbing for female patients. Greasy skin and acne are accompanying features.

D TRUE Nystagmus, ataxia, diplopia and vertigo, are the outcome of the cerebellar vestibular dysfunction produced by phenytoin.

E TRUE Gingival hyperplasia occurs in about 20 per cent of patients during chronic therapy with phenytoin and is one of the commonest manifestations of toxicity in young patients. It is apparently the result of altered collagen metabolism. The effects can be kept to a minimum by good oral hygiene.

185 The anaesthetic thiopentone

    A produces analgesia
    B may cause necrosis when given intravenously as a 2.5 per cent solution
    C has a short duration of action because it is rapidly metabolised
    D is a barbiturate
    E may cause laryngospasm

A FALSE Thiopentone is not analgesic, indeed low doses may be antianalgesic, and when used by itself the unconscious patient may react to painful stimuli.

B FALSE For induction of anaesthesia thiopentone is normally given intravenously and whilst injection of 5 per cent solution into small veins may cause thrombosis, when using 2.5 per cent solution tissue necrosis is only likely if extravasation or inadvertent intra-arterial injection occurs. The arterial spasm following the latter may then be sufficiently severe to induce gangrene.

C FALSE Thiopentone is a highly lipid soluble drug, and is rapidly taken up into brain tissue to produce its anaesthetic action. As the blood concentration falls it leaks out of the brain back into the blood and consciousness is restored. Redistribution into adipose tissue elsewhere in the body, by maintaining the low blood level, ensures continued recovery.

D TRUE Thiopentone is the sulphur analogue of pentobarbitone. Such thiobarbiturates are more lipid soluble and have a more rapid onset and shorter duration of action than the corresponding oxybarbiturate (see C).

E TRUE Apnoea, coughing, laryngospasm and bronchospasm are not uncommon complications of thiopentone use.

186 Typically induction of anaesthesia with

    A trichloroethylene is accompanied by useful analgesia

    B thiopentone (2.5 per cent) in a fit adult takes about 2 minutes

    C methohexitone produces unconsciousness for longer than with thiopentone

    D ether is pleasant

    E halothane is effected with 10 per cent by volume in combination with oxygen and nitrous oxide (25 : 75)

A TRUE Although a relatively weak anaesthetic, trichloroethylene is a strong analgesic, and self-administration apparatus enables it to be used in midwifery to control labour pains.

B FALSE Anaesthesia following intravenous injection of 2.5 per cent thiopentone is effected in a fit adult within about 10 to 15 seconds without a clinically obvious excitement phase. However, in children (where only 1 per cent is used) and in frail old ladies where the drug is given deliberately slowly, induction may take 2 minutes.

C FALSE Methohexitone is 2.5 to 3 times more potent than thiopentone, and immediate recovery of consciousness is more rapid than with thiopentone. This relates to the lower binding to plasma protein, the higher proportion that is unionised at body pH, and the consequent ease of movement in and out of body lipids.

D FALSE Ether has a pungent odour and at concentrations required for induction of anaesthesia is extremely irritant to mucous membranes, causing increased salivary and bronchial secretions. This and its high solubility in blood mean that induction is both prolonged and extremely unpleasant, and may be followed by a long excitement phase.

E FALSE Halothane is a very potent anaesthetic and induction of anaesthesia is normally carried out by passing a mixture of oxygen and nitrous oxide (in the ratio by volume of 25 : 75) through a vaporiser so that 2 to 4 per cent halothane is added. For maintenance of anaesthesia, this is reduced to between 0.5 per cent and 2 per cent.

187 Which of the following statements is/are true

    A trichloroethylene should not be used in a closed circuit
    B halothane relaxes the uterus
    C nitrous oxide and oxygen 80 : 20 gives good muscular relaxation
    D ether is relatively insoluble in blood
    E halothane is a gas at room temperature

A TRUE Trichloroethylene is broken down when drawn over the soda lime in a closed circuit system, and the breakdown products have a selective toxic action on the trigeminal nerve.

B TRUE Halothane strongly inhibits myometrial tone which means that it should be employed with caution during delivery.

C FALSE 100 per cent nitrous oxide used to be used to produce 'secondary saturation' a cyanotic condition which causes excellent muscular relaxation for abdominal surgery. However, this procedure is dangerous and has been discontinued. When given in the absence of hypoxia or other drugs nitrous oxide does not induce muscle relaxation.

D FALSE Solubility of an anaesthetic in blood is usually expressed as the blood : gas partition coefficient or λ, which represents the ratio of anaesthetic concentration in blood to the anaesthetic concentration in the gas phase when the two are in equilibrium. The more soluble the anaesthetic in blood, the more of it must be dissolved in blood to raise its partial pressure, and the more slowly anaesthesia is induced. Ether is very soluble in blood with a blood : gas partition coefficient of 12, and consequently induction is prolonged.

E FALSE At room temperature, halothane is a volatile liquid. It is administered from a vaporiser by bubbling through it oxygen and nitrous oxide gases.

188 Halothane is extensively used because in addition to being a good anaesthetic, it

    A may be administered safely by unskilled personnel
    B produces excellent relaxation of abdominal muscles
    C has a potent analgesic action
    D is not irritant
    E is without toxicity to the heart

A FALSE Possibly the most important danger in the use of halothane is its extreme potency. Anaesthesia may be induced in a few minutes with just 2 to 4 per cent and if the concentration is not reduced the patient will pass rapidly through the planes of anaesthesia and into cardiac and respiratory depression. Less potent anaesthetics like ether are much more easily controlled by the unskilled.

B FALSE Halothane produces excellent relaxation of the jaw so that intubation can easily be performed using only this. However, muscular relaxation as a whole is poor, and although deepening anaesthesia enables better relaxation to be achieved, a neuromuscular blocker would normally be given in preference to relax abdominal muscles.

C FALSE It has no useful analgesic potential of its own and is normally given with nitrous oxide which is a good analgesic.

D TRUE Unlike ether which was the most widely used anaesthetic before the introduction of halothane, it is not irritant to mucous membranes.

E FALSE As with most anaesthetics the blood pressure falls with deepening anaesthesia; but in addition halothane sensitises the myocardium to catecholamines, especially adrenaline, which can provoke severe dysrhythmias. This property is common to many halogenated hydrocarbons.

189 Nitrous oxide and oxygen (50 : 50)

    A produces good anaesthesia
    B produces good analgesia
    C is a useful agent to give to patients following myocardial infarction
    D causes uterine relaxation
    E is inflammable

A FALSE Nitrous oxide is a weak anaesthetic, and even at the highest concentration at which adequate oxygenation is maintained, i.e. 80 per cent nitrous oxide : 20 per cent oxygen, it is impossible to achieve adequate anaesthesia.

B TRUE Nitrous oxide is a useful analgesic and cylinders of oxygen and nitrous oxide (50 : 50) are standard equipment for ambulances to provide analgesia and sedation for patients in pain travelling to hospital (see C). At concentrations between 50 per cent to 80 per cent some studies indicate that nitrous oxide is a comparable analgesic to morphine.

C TRUE When administered as indicated in B, nitrous oxide is very useful for controlling the pain and allaying the anxiety associated with myocardial infarction. However, its use has been questioned recently following the finding that nitrous oxide depresses cardiac contractility.

D FALSE Nitrous oxide is commonly administered in obstetric practice for its analgesic action, and at 50 : 50 combination with oxygen alters neither uterine function nor maternal blood oxygenation.

E FALSE Nitrous oxide and oxygen is neither inflammable nor explosive, but it will support combustion.

190 Surgical anaesthesia induced with ether is

A rapid
B accompanied by good muscle relaxation
C accompanied by increased myocardial excitability
D associated with a higher incidence of hepatitis than with other anaesthetics
E dangerous because of the risk of explosion

A FALSE Both induction and recovery from ether anaesthesia are prolonged. This is largely because ether is highly soluble in blood and the rise in gas partial pressure is slow.

B TRUE Muscle relaxation during surgical anaesthesia is good, and ether is satisfactory for abdominal surgery. Its action is partly due to cns depression, and partly by direct action on the end plate.

C FALSE Ether neither increases myocardial excitability nor causes cardiac dysrhythmias.

D FALSE Following surgical operations, there is a minute incidence of hepatic disease due to infections or serum hepatitis. However, there is no evidence that ether contributes to this incidence, although during its administration ether does depress liver function.

E TRUE Ether is inflammable and in combination with oxygen forms an explosive mixture. Ant-static equipment is necessary to reduce the possibility of a spark and diathermy cannot be carried out. When ether was widely used there were many accidents.

191 Which of the following is/are true

  A hypoxia may occur after administration of nitrous oxide has ceased
  B gases with high solubility in blood induce anaesthesia rapidly
  C cyclopropane is administered in a closed circuit
  D althesin is a mixture of two barbiturate anaesthetics
  E after two hours of anaesthesia the arterial blood tension of nitrous
     oxide is less than 10 per cent of the tension in the inspired gas

---

A TRUE When nitrous oxide anaesthesia ceases, the nitrous oxide in the blood escapes into the lungs very rapidly. This has the effect of diluting the oxygen and reducing the alveolar oxygen concentration. The phenomenon is known as diffusion hypoxia, and although rarely a danger can be avoided by administering oxygen for a few minutes at the end of the anaesthesia.

B FALSE With a given gaseous anaesthetic, the depth of anaesthesia is determined by the partial pressure of anaesthetic agent in the brain, and in turn, therefore on the partial pressure of the agent in the blood. The greater the solubility of the agent in blood, the more of it must be dissolved in order to raise its partial pressure, and the more slowly, therefore, anaesthesia is induced.

C TRUE Cyclopropane is inflammable and explosive and in order to achieve safety (and economy) it requires a closed or semi-closed system.

D FALSE Althesin is a mixture of two steroids based on the pregnane nucleus, alphaxolone and alphadolone in the ratio 3 : 1. Alphadolone has only half the anaesthetic activity of alphaxolone but is necessary to enhance the solubility of alphaxolone. They are dissolved in Cremophor EL (polyoxyethylated castor oil).

E FALSE Nitrous oxide is poorly soluble in blood (see B), and its tension in arteriolar blood reaches 90 per cent of the inspired tension within about 20 minutes of the start of anaesthesia.

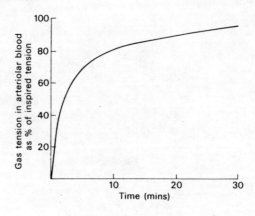

192 Enkephalin

    A is a pentapeptide
    B is found primarily in the pituitary
    C binds to opiate receptors but is not antagonised by naloxone
    D has a prolonged action in the brain
    E is also known as endorphin

A TRUE In 1975 two naturally occurring pentapeptides were discovered in the brain which were shown to bind to morphine receptors. They have been called methionine- and leucine-enkephalin and have the following structures:

    Met-enkephalin   Met-Phe-Gly-Gly-Tyr
    Leu-enkephalin   Leu-Phe-Gly-Gly-Tyr

B FALSE The enkephalins are found in the cns primarily in the striatum and hypothalamus. It is endorphins that are found mainly in the pituitary (see E).

C FALSE The property of enkephalins to bind to opiate receptors throughout the body and to have their actions antagonised by naloxone provided part of the initial evidence to support the existence of these substances.

D FALSE Amino- and carboxy-peptidases present in the brain rapidly destroy enkephalins to limit their duration of action.

E FALSE Endorphin is the name which has been given to the larger naturally occurring polypeptides which are found in the pituitary and which derive from the pituitary peptide β-lipotropin. The various polypeptides are shown below. They all include amino acid residues 61 to 65 (which is met-enkephalin).

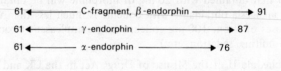

61 ◄——————— C-fragment, β-endorphin ——————► 91
61 ◄——————— γ-endorphin ——————► 87
61 ◄——— α-endorphin ——————► 76

61 ◄— met-enkephalin —► 65

193 In the choice of an analgesic for the treatment of acute clinical pain, which of the following statements is/are true

    A pethidine is suitable for use in labour because it does not depress the respiration of the fetus

    B pholcodine is a superior analgesic to codeine

    C phenazocine is weight for weight a more potent analgesic than morphine

    D 240 mg of codeine produces equivalent analgesia to 20 mg of morphine

    E dihydrocodeine is a Schedule II drug (both in the UK and the USA) and as such its prescription is restricted in the same way as with morphine

---

A FALSE Pethidine in common with other narcotic analgesics causes respiratory depression, and if given to pregnant women during labour will cross the placenta into the fetus. If the time between administration of the drug and delivery of the baby is long ($>$ 1 hour) then sufficient pethidine may enter the fetal circulation to produce significant respiratory depression. Pethidine does not appear to alter uterine contractility or to increase the incidence of postpartum haemorrhage.

B FALSE Pholcodine is a synthetic morphine derivative with little, if any, analgesic activity, but with significant antitussive action. It causes less constipation than codeine and is well tolerated by children.

C TRUE As an analgesic, phenazocine is some 3 to 5 times more potent than morphine, and has a more prolonged action.

D FALSE Morphine is about 12 times more potent than codeine. However, that does not mean that by increasing the dose of codeine to 240 mg an equivalent level of analgesia to that obtained with 20 mg of morphine will be obtained. The maximum level of analgesia obtainable with codeine is much less than with morphine, and even at doses of about 100 mg codeine causes unpleasant toxicity (abdominal pain, nausea, vomiting, sedation, etc.).

E FALSE Schedule II of the Misuse of Drugs Act in the UK and of the Controlled Substances Act in the USA restricts the production, supply and prescription of certain substances. Addictive drugs like morphine, pethidine and methadone fall into this category. Dihydrocodeine on which dependence is rare falls into Schedule I in the UK and Schedule III in the USA. Normal prescription of dihydrocodeine for medical reasons is thus permitted.

194 Following dental surgery a patient receives an intravenous injection of what may or may not be an opiate analgesic. Neither the patient nor the operator know that it is actually saline. The alleviation of pain that results

    A is known as a placebo response
    B is due to prostaglandin release at the site of surgery
    C may be blocked by naloxone
    D will not be improved by subsequent administration of morphine
    E is accompanied by respiratory depression

A TRUE Placebo is Latin for 'I please' and the placebo response refers to the improvement of a patient's condition following administration of an inert dummy tablet or an injection of saline. The effect is thought to be a psychological response to the interest shown by the doctor, and the suggestion instilled in the patient that treatment will be beneficial. Many factors are involved, including the colour of the tablet, the doctors' powers of persuasion, and the patient's belief, conscious or otherwise, that the therapy will be effective.

B FALSE On the contrary, release of prostaglandins at a site of injury and inflammation will potentiate the pain response that occurs. Pain-producing agents like bradykinin and histamine have been shown to have more marked algesic actions in the presence of prostaglandins. Indeed the analgesic action of drugs like aspirin is primarily due to their ability to reduce the local synthesis of prostaglandins in such a reaction.

C TRUE Naloxone is a competitive antagonist of morphine and other opiates, and experimental studies have shown that if it is given to a patient who has benefited from a placebo, the pain will become more intense. It has been suggested that this is due to the ability of naloxone to prevent the action of enkephalins released within the cns as part of the normal reaction to pain.

D FALSE Although alleviation of pain will occur following saline injection except in a few highly susceptible individuals, this is rarely of sufficient intensity to completely control the pain. Morphine will increase the pain threshold and reduce the awareness of pain still further.

E FALSE Unless the subject in such a trial is familiar with the side effects of morphine, then effects resembling the toxic actions of morphine are not likely to occur.

195 In the clinical management of pain

A nalorphine is the drug of choice for the treatment of respiratory depression due to morphine overdose

B pethidine overdose is characterised by pin-point pupils

C due to chronic conditions like rheumatoid arthritis, methadone is an
excellent alternative if indomethacin fails to produce adequate analgesia

D methadone is less addicting than morphine

E dihydrocodeine is less potent than codeine

A FALSE Nalorphine is a partial antagonist at the opiate receptor site which means that not only will it overcome the effects of morphine and related drugs, but it may in its own right produce morphine-like actions. This confuses its use and although it was once used to treat morphine poisoning, it has since been replaced by the pure antagonist naloxone.

B FALSE The morphine-like action of the synthetic drug, pethidine, was dis-covered by accident during a search for a muscarinic blocker. It is a piperidine molecule and its main action is as a central analgesic, but it has measurable atropine-like activity. This is of little clinical significance except that in overdose it causes pupillary dilatation, rather than the pin-point pupils seen with morphine.

C FALSE Although methadone is less addicting than morphine (see D), it still has strong euphoriant and dependence-producing properties. It would, therefore, be inappropriate therapy in a chronic non-fatal condition which could continue for many years. Supplementation of the indomethacin with aspirin, paracetamol, codeine or even dihydrocodeine would be the correct course.

D TRUE Prolonged use of methadone can lead to dependence of the morphine type but it is milder and thought to be easier to treat than morphine addiction. For this reason, methadone has found a role as substitution therapy in morphine and heroin addicts.

E FALSE Dihydrocodeine has approximately twice the analgesic effect of codeine, and is unlikely to cause dependence. It provides an excellent treatment for moderately severe ongoing pain.

196 Which of the following statements about the narcotic analgesics is/are correct

A codeine has useful antitussive properties
B codeine has useful antipyretic properties
C pentazocine is less addicting than morphine
D pentazocine may cause hallucinations
E morphine is used to control diarrhoea

A TRUE Cough suppression is a feature of the opiates and is due to a direct action on the cough centre of the brain. Codeine is widely used because it produces less respiratory depression, nausea and vomiting than morphine. It also has little addictive potential.

B FALSE In common with other opiates, codeine does not possess antipyretic activity. Drugs like aspirin which do possess this action are inhibitors of prostaglandin synthesis, and this is not a property of codeine (see question 124, page 145).

C TRUE On a weight basis pentazocine has about one third the analgesic potency of morphine. It also produces less euphoria than morphine and large doses cause hallucinations and anxiety. This means that it is less enjoyable to take and addiction is less likely. The exclusion of this drug from Schedule II of the Misuse of Drugs Act in the UK and Schedule II of the Controlled Substances Act in the USA reflects its lower addicting potential.

D TRUE Hallucinations and anxiety may be produced by large doses of pentazocine. This is known as a dysphoric reaction, and is similar to that seen with nalorphine.

E TRUE Morphine and its derivatives all bind to a greater or lesser extent to specific receptors on the smooth muscle of the gastrointestinal tract. The effect is to increase the tone of the muscle and to reduce peristaltic contractions. This is of value in the treatment of diarrhoea, where gastrointestinal propulsive activity is increased. Morphine is given in small amounts (< 1 mg) often in combination with agents that increase the viscosity of the gut contents (e.g. kaolin).

221

197 Dextropropoxyphene

A is chemically related to methadone
B has similar analgesic potency to pethidine
C when given with paracetamol provides a useful anti-inflammatory analgesic combination
D in overdose causes death due to hepatotoxicity
E is not addictive

A TRUE Dextropropoxyphene is the D(+) isomer of propoxyphene and is chemically related to methadone.

$$CH_3CH_2C - O - C - CH - CH_2 - N \quad CH_3/CH_3$$

propoxyphene   methadone

B FALSE Most evidence suggests that dextropropoxyphene, if it has useful analgesic activity at all, is of similar potency to codeine and that the maximum degree of analgesia that can be obtained with it is only a fraction of that which can be produced with pethidine.

C FALSE Neither paracetamol nor dextropropoxyphene have anti-inflammatory properties and although this drug combination as Distalgesic is frequently used in conditions in which inflammation is an important component (e.g. rheumatic diseases, toothache, etc.) its usefulness is entirely due to its analgesic action (but see B).

D FALSE Overdosage with dextropropoxyphene produces a picture similar to that seen with other opiate analgesics. This includes cardiac and respiratory depression leading to coma and convulsions. Hepatotoxicity is not seen except when the drug has been consumed in combination with paracetamol as Distalgesic. In the UK this is currently one of the commonest causes of death from drug overdosage.

E FALSE Although dextropropoxyphene is only mildly euphoriant, and high doses or parenteral administration may cause psychotic reactions, it is still addictive. The potential for abuse is much less than with morphine or pethidine, but addiction still occurs.

198 Morphine

   A is a metabolite of codeine
   B may cause vomiting
   C may cause diarrhoea
   D has specific receptors in the cns
   E has specific receptors in the gastrointestinal tract

A TRUE Codeine is methyl morphine and has about one twelfth of the potency of morphine. About 10 per cent of administered codeine is demethylated to morphine and free and conjugated morphine can be found in the urine following therapeutic doses of codeine. To what extent this morphine contributes to the effects of codeine is unclear, but it would appear to be small since when the amount of administered codeine is increased it is never possible to obtain the same degree of analgesia as produced by morphine.

B TRUE Morphine stimulates the chemoreceptor trigger zone (ctz) in the area postrema of the medulla, causing vomiting in about one third of ambulatory patients. It occurs less readily in patients confined to bed suggesting that a vestibular component is also important.

C FALSE By an action directly on receptors in the smooth muscle throughout the gastrointestinal tract, morphine and other opiates increase the tone of the smooth muscle and reduce the propulsive contractions, consequently slowing the movement of the gut contents. This action, particularly in the colon, causes dessication of the faeces and constipation. Opiates are thus very useful in controlling severe diarrhoea, e.g. in dysentery.

D TRUE It has been known for many years that specific opiate receptors exist in certain areas of the brain, and that morphine and related analgesics bind to these sites in order to produce their pharmacological effects. The true significance of these receptors has been realised only recently with the discovery of naturally occurring peptides, called enkephalins, which also bind to these receptors. The action of both morphine and the enkephalins in the cns are inhibited by the specific antagonist, naloxone.

E TRUE The actions of morphine on the gastrointestinal tract (see C) are due to binding of morphine to specific receptors on the smooth muscle, and as with the central actions of morphine can be blocked by the use of the specific antagonist naloxone. The presence of specific receptors to morphine in this easily isolated tissue has contributed greatly to the investigation of the enkephalins and endorphins.

199 Morphine is useful in the clinical treatment of

    A biliary colic
    B gastrointestinal obstruction
    C cardiac asthma
    D terminal cancer pain
    E chronic respiratory disease

A FALSE After therapeutic doses of morphine the pressure in the biliary tract can increase tenfold from less than 20 mm of H_2O to in excess of 200 mm of H_2O. This may by itself be sufficient to induce epigastric pain similar to biliary colic, and in patients with this condition morphine is contraindicated. The rise in biliary pressure is due to contraction of the smooth muscle of the sphincter of Oddi.

B FALSE Morphine causes a rise in the resting tone of the smooth muscle throughout the gastrointestinal tract and a reduction in the amplitude of propulsive contractions. The overall effect is a constipating one which would complicate obstruction.

C TRUE Cardiac asthma is the name given to bouts of paroxysmal nocturnal dyspnoea which may follow left ventricular failure. It is due to the pulmonary congestion and oedema that occurs when lying flat. The patient has a sense of suffocation, is fighting for breath, and in severe attacks may cough up frothy blood-stained sputum. Morphine rapidly relieves such attacks, but the mechanism is unclear and may simply be removal of fear and apprehension. Morphine is generally contraindicated when respiration is impaired (see E).

D TRUE Opiate analgesics should generally not be used in treating *chronic* painful conditions because the patients become addicted and develop tolerance to the drug. The one exception is the treatment of pain associated with terminal diseases, especially cancer. In addition to the pain relief the euphoria and tranquillity produced by the drug are of particular help to the patient.

E FALSE Morphine reduces the responsiveness of the respiratory centre to increases in carbon dioxide tension (PCO_2). This result is a reduction in respiratory rate, minute volume and tidal exchange. This combined with its ability in some patients to cause mast cell degranulation and thus induce bronchoconstriction, means that morphine is contraindicated in any diseases where respiratory function is chronically impaired, e.g. asthma, bronchitis (but see C).

200 Which of the following may occur as a complication of morphine treatment of acute pain

    A addiction
    B antihistaminic effects
    C a rise in systemic arterial blood pressure
    D constriction of smooth muscle sphincters
    E stimulation of the respiratory centre

A FALSE Although many addicts claim that they were 'hooked' following a single injection of morphine or heroin, this is not the clinical picture and addiction does not interfere with the treatment of acute pain. Only following repeated administration over a period of time would this present a problem, and except in terminal cases morphine should not be used in this way.

B FALSE Morphine is a base and will release histamine from mast cells. Locally this will cause itching and systemically may provoke a fall in blood pressure (see C), and bronchoconstriction.

C FALSE Therapeutic doses of morphine have little effect on blood pressure or heart rate in the supine patient, but if the patient sits up, orthostatic hypotension and fainting may occur. It is the result of peripheral vasodilation, partly due to histamine release (see B) and partly by another undefined mechanism.

D TRUE Morphine increases the tone of smooth muscle and as a result the sphincters in the urinary bladder and bile duct (sphincter of Oddi) will be contracted. The effect on the former is to cause urinary retention (despite increasing tone of the detrusor muscle of the bladder) and on the latter to increase the pressure in the biliary duct which may aggravate biliary colic.

E FALSE Morphine, even within the therapeutic range, has a progressive depressant action on the respiratory centres, decreasing both the rate and depth of respiration. Reduced responsiveness of the centres to an increase in carbon dioxide tension (PCO_2), appears to be the mechanism involved.

201 Diamorphine (heroin)

    A is converted in the body to morphine
    B causes nausea and vomiting
    C is a respiratory depressant
    D causes pin-point pupils
    E has potent atropine-like properties

A TRUE Heroin is rapidly hydrolysed to monoacetyl morphine which in turn is hydrolysed to morphine. Most of the evidence suggests that the morphine is responsible for the pharmacological actions of heroin.

B TRUE Nausea and vomiting are characteristic of heroin usage and are largely the result of direct stimulation of the chemoreceptor trigger zone; although a greater action on ambulant compared with bedridden patients suggests a vestibular action as well. Addicts describe this effect of heroin as 'good sick' because it precedes the euphoriant actions of the drug.

C TRUE As with other opiates heroin is a respiratory depressant, reducing the responsiveness of the brain stem respiratory centres to the stimulant effects of carbon dioxide tension (PCO_2).

D TRUE Pin-point pupils are characteristic of opiate abuse. It is due to stimulation of the IIIrd nerve nucleus, the nerves from which supply the constrictor pupillae of the iris. Mydriasis produced by asphyxia (for example following inhalation of vomit) may, however, confuse this diagnosis.

E FALSE Of the common opioid analgesics only the synthetic agent pethidine has significant atropine-like activity.

202 Naloxone

A is analgesic
B causes euphoria
C is the drug of first choice for the treatment of opiate overdose
D is a partial agonist for the opiate receptor
E causes a withdrawal syndrome if given to an opiate-dependent subject

---

A FALSE Naloxone is a pure antagonist of morphine (see D) and as such has no morphine-like activity itself. It does not therefore cause analgesia, respiratory depression, constipation or euphoria.

B FALSE See A.

C TRUE Because naloxone is a pure antagonist and free from morphine-like activity, it is the drug of choice in the treatment of overdose from any opiate, i.e. morphine, heroin, pethidine, pentazocine, dextropropoxyphene, etc.

D FALSE A partial agonist is a drug which on contact with receptors initially stimulates them, but because it dissociates slowly from the receptor it acts as an antagonist to other agonists. The morphine antagonist, nalorphine is such a drug, but naloxone is a pure antagonist (see A).

E TRUE By abolishing the dependence-producing effects of morphine and related compounds, naloxone will, if given to an addict, precipitate a withdrawal syndrome.

203 In the relief of pain in advanced malignant disease

A anti-inflammatory analgesics like aspirin are ineffective

B narcotic analgesics will only produce adequate analgesia if given by injection

C diazepam is a useful adjunct to therapy because it controls the nausea and vomiting induced by the opiate analgesics

D only morphine or more potent agents of the same type will control the pain due to bone metastases

E constipation is a complicating feature of opiate usage

A FALSE A recognised principle in the treatment of the chronic progressing pain of terminal diseases is that potent narcotic analgesics like morphine should be reserved for use when all else fails, and that at the outset many patients will obtain relief with aspirin. High doses are required (up to 1200 mg every four to six hours) and intolerance or poor compliance may be a problem. In this case, benorylate suspension (an ester of aspirin and paracetamol) which is better tolerated may be preferable.

B FALSE Morphine and related analgesics are indeed more potent when given by injection, but most patients can be maintained very successfully on oral medication. Both morphine and diamorphine can be given over a wide dosage range (5 to 100 mg every 4 hours) and only if, despite giving an antiemetic, nausea and vomiting persist should parenteral administration be used.

C FALSE Pain is not simply the recognition by the cns of a set of electrical impulses travelling to the brain; it is a complex and highly subjective emotional reaction to that information. Fear and anxiety play a large part in aggravating pain, and anxiolytic drugs like diazepam may help to reduce the amount of analgesic required. Diazepam does not control nausea and vomiting. If necessary this can be achieved with antiemetics such as prochlorperazine.

D FALSE Pain in bones responds only poorly to morphine-like analgesics and where bone metastases are a source of pain, non-steroidal anti-inflammatory drugs (e.g. aspirin, phenylbutazone) or radiotherapy should be considered.

E TRUE Opiates act on the gastrointestinal tract to increase the tone of the smooth muscle and to reduce the propulsive contractions. This action, particularly on the colon, will over a period of time, cause dessication of the faeces and constipation. Mild faecal-softening laxatives may be required.

204 Ethyl alcohol

    A is excreted unchanged in alveolar air
    B may cause cutaneous vasoconstriction
    C antagonises the effects of barbiturate hypnotics
    D elimination from the bloodstream follows an exponential curve, i.e. first order kinetics
    E is excreted almost entirely unchanged

A TRUE The concentration of ethyl alcohol in alveolar air is about 0.05 per cent of that in the blood, and this provides the basis of the 'breathalyser'. However, the loss of alcohol in the expired air even together with that excreted in the urine only constitutes about 2 per cent of ingested alcohol. A severely intoxicated individual with a blood alcohol of 400 mg per cent will lose about 200 mg of alcohol/100 l of expired air.

B FALSE Vasodilatation normally follows consumption of moderate amounts of alcohol to produce a warm flushed skin. It is most probably a result of central depression of the cardiovascular centre. Although it produces a warm sensation, it is unwise to use alcohol as fortification against extreme cold, since loss of body heat occurs more readily. This has undoubtedly contributed to many acute alcohol deaths.

C FALSE Both ethyl alcohol and the barbiturates are progressive depressants of cns function, and as such the action of alcohol is at least additive with that of the barbiturates, and may even potentiate their effect. The most important aspect of this interaction is that the lethal dose of the barbiturates is reduced in the presence of alcohol. Many deaths or near deaths result annually from this combination.

D FALSE The metabolism of alcohol differs from most other substances in that the rate of oxidation does not increase as the concentration in the blood increases, i.e. zero order kinetics apply. Thus the amount of alcohol metabolised per unit time is constant for a single individual and roughly proportional to their body weight (and more importantly to liver weight). The average rate of metabolism is about 10 ml ethanol/hour.

E FALSE About 98 per cent of consumed ethanol is metabolised, primarily in the liver, and only about 2 per cent is excreted unchanged (see A).

205 Ethyl alcohol

    A initially stimulates then depresses the cns
    B reduces the release of antidiuretic hormone (ADH) from the pituitary
    C can be used to treat the 'acetaldehyde syndrome' associated with disul-
       firam
    D increases the ratio of NADH : NAD in the liver
    E antagonises the gastric bleeding due to aspirin

A FALSE Alcohol has a direct progressive depressant action on the cns. The apparent stimulation produced initially is due to the unrestrained activity of certain areas of the brain from which inhibitory control has been removed.

B TRUE Although the large amounts of fluid commonly ingested in alcoholic drinks undoubtedly increase urine production, alcohol also enhances diuresis by decreasing tubular reabsorption of water. The mechanism is indirect. Alcohol acts on the neurohypophysis to inhibit the release of ADH which in turn has a reduced effect on the collecting ducts in the medullary portion of the kidney, so that urine output increases.

C FALSE Disulfiram is used in aversion therapy for the treatment of alcoholics. It competes with NAD^+ for sites on the acetaldehyde dehydrogenase enzyme and so halts metabolism of ethyl alcohol at the aldehyde stage (see D). As the acetaldehyde accumulates in the body, flushing, nausea, vomiting and headaches occur; signs and symptoms known as the 'acetaldehyde syndrome'.

D TRUE The oxidation of alcohol in the liver occurs mainly in two steps, both of which utilise NAD^+ as the hydrogen acceptor.

$$C_2H_5OH + NAD^+ \xrightarrow[\text{dehydrogenase}]{\text{alcohol}} CH_3CHO + NADH + H^+$$

$$CH_3CHO + NAD^+ + CoASH \xrightarrow[\text{dehydrogenase}]{\text{aldehyde}} CH_3COSCoA + NADH + H^+$$
$$\text{acetyl CoA}$$

The effect is to increase the ratio of NADH : NAD in the liver, which in turn causes metabolic changes such as hyperuricaemia, enhanced fatty acid and lactate production and reduced gluconeogenesis.

E FALSE The effect of ethanol by itself on the stomach depends on the concentration. Below 20 per cent it stimulates gastric secretions, above 20 per cent it inhibits secretions, and above 40 per cent it may induce gastritis. In any event it appears to enhance the gastric toxicity of aspirin, and bleeding may be made worse.

206 Ethanol metabolism

    A occurs to a large extent in the gastric mucosa
    B is effected by liver cell microsomal enzymes
    C is effected by liver cell cytosol enzymes
    D follows zero order kinetics
    E produces about 2 Kcal/g

A FALSE Ethanol is absorbed from and secreted into the stomach through the gastric mucosa, but there is no evidence for significant metabolism in this tissue. The majority of alcohol degradation ($>$ 90 per cent) occurs in the liver.

B TRUE The main pathway for metabolism of alcohol involves liver cell cytosol enzymes (see C), but a small proportion is also oxidised by the non-specific microsomal drug metabolising system in the liver.

$$C_2H_5OH + NADPH + H^+ + O_2 \longrightarrow CH_3CHO + NADP^+ + 2H_2O$$

This sytem becomes of greater importance in subjects in whom enzymes have been induced by previous chronic consumption of drugs such as barbiturates or even ethanol.

C TRUE Oxidation of ethanol to acetaldehyde is primarily catalysed by alcohol dehydrogenase found in the cytosol of hepatic cells.

$$C_2H_5OH + NAD^+ \longrightarrow CH_3CHO + NADH + H^+$$

D TRUE The metabolism of alcohol differs from that of most substances in that the rate of oxidation does not increase as the substrate concentration increases. In other words zero order kinetics apply, the rate of oxidation being roughly proportional to the body weight (or more importantly to liver weight) of the individual. The average rate of metabolism is about 10 ml/hour.

E FALSE Alcohol is a quickly absorbed and immediately available source of energy, releasing about 7 Kcal/g (29 KJ/g). The average daily consumption of alcohol in Western countries means that it contributes significantly to the daily food intake.

207 Which of the following statements about ethyl alcohol is/are true

    A in Britain 70° proof whisky contains about 25 per cent alcohol (v/v)

    B the rate of absorption from the gastrointestinal tract is maximal at a concentration of about 20 per cent

    C the legal limit for driving a car in Britain is 80 mg per cent ethyl alcohol in blood

    D two hours after an alcoholic drink the urine level of alcohol will usually be slightly higher than the blood level

    E most people are obviously inebriated at blood levels of 30 mg per cent

---

A FALSE In Britain proof spirit contains 57.1 per cent v/v or 49.2 per cent w/w ethyl alcohol. The strength of alcoholic beverages may be expressed in terms of the degrees of proof where proof spirit is designated 100°. Thus whisky which is 70° proof may also be described as 30° underproof and contains about 40 per cent v/v ethyl alcohol. In the USA proof spirit contains less alcohol (50 per cent v/v).

B TRUE Alcohol taken orally is rapidly absorbed from both the stomach and small intestine and, as might be expected, up to a certain point the higher the concentration of alcohol imbibed the more rapidly the blood level rises, peak rates of absorption occurring with aperitifs — sherry and vermouth — which contain about 20 per cent alcohol. Above this level slowed gastric emptying, pyloric spasm and perhaps gastritis will delay absorption. The presence of food will impair absorption throughout the concentration range.

C TRUE The Road Safety Act 1967 made it an offence in Britain to drive a car with a blood level of ethyl alcohol in excess of 80 mg/100 ml or a urine level of more than 107 mg/ml.

D TRUE Although alcohol is largely metabolised by the liver and negligible amounts are excreted in the urine (normal about 2 per cent), the absolute concentration of alcohol in the urine following a single alcoholic drink will usually be slightly higher than the blood level, and perhaps as much as 20 per cent higher. This is because the appearance of alcohol in the urine is dependent on the blood alcohol level, but once in the urine (unlike that in the blood) it is not available for metabolism.

E FALSE It is possible to demonstrate experimentally threshold effects such as increased reaction time, diminished fine motor control and impaired critical faculties with concentrations of ethyl alcohol in blood as low as 20 to 30 mg per cent. However, most individuals are not obviously inebriated and would not be so until they reach 50 to 100 mg per cent and experienced drinkers can often conceal their intoxication at levels considerably in excess of this (> 150 mg per cent).

208 Ethyl alcohol

A can cause mental symptoms when withdrawn from chronic drinkers
B can cause mental symptoms due to organic brain damage
C potentiates the sedative action of amitryptyline
D can aggravate Parkinsonism
E withdrawal from an alcoholic can aggravate epilepsy

A **TRUE** In addition to tremor, nausea and sweating, withdrawal of alcohol from a chronic alcoholic will initially cause anxiety, but as hallucinations develop a true psychosis will reveal itself.

B **TRUE** A psychosis is termed organic when there is a specific identifiable cause, e.g. alcohol abuse, and in some chronic conditions where there are associated histopathological changes. Degeneration in the cerebellum and corpus callosum occurs in some alcoholics but the aetiology is not clear. Poor nutrition and vitamin deficiency complicate the picture further. The outcome is a complex psychiatric state which may include dementia, hallucinations of the schizophrenic type, and paranoia.

C **TRUE** Alcohol is a cns depressant the action of which progresses as the dose increases, eventually causing hypnosis. Although amitryptiline is an antidepressant it also has mild tranquillising properties and the most common side effect is drowsiness. Alcohol potentiates this action of amitryptiline and the combination could prove dangerous.

D **FALSE** Although many drugs (e.g. phenothiazines) by interfering with dopamine metabolism can provoke Parkinsonian symptoms, and thus complicate treatment of the disease, this is not a feature of ethyl alcohol. The tremors seen in alcoholics following withdrawal may, however, be mistaken for Parkinsonism.

E **TRUE** Withdrawal of alcohol from a chronic drinker may provoke a seizure of the grand mal type.

209 Withdrawal of alcohol from a dependent individual may produce

    A goose pimples and shivering
    B anxiety
    C sleepiness
    D tremor
    E convulsions

A FALSE Goose pimples and shivering (cold turkey) are a characteristic of withdrawal from opiates, not alcohol.

B TRUE Characteristically, alcohol-dependent subjects who abstain from drinking will show severe anxiety, weakness, sweating, nausea and perhaps vomiting. They hallucinate, commonly 'seeing' insects rather than the much caricatured pink elephants, and have tremors which are often so severe that they cannot even hold a glass (see also C, D, E).

C FALSE Alcohol has an hypnotic action and during its withdrawal alcoholics are restless and anxious. They 'see' things at first only when their eyes are closed and they are often so terrified that they are reluctant even to try to sleep. A rebound increase in the proportion of rem (dream) sleep during withdrawal may aggravate this.

D TRUE The tremulous state during withdrawal (see B) reaches a peak within 24 to 48 hours after stopping drinking and when accompanied by severe hallucinations produces the state given the general term *delirium tremens.*

E TRUE Grand mal seizures may occur following alcohol withdrawal although they are less common than following barbiturate withdrawal. They are most likely to occur in the first 24 hours.

210 Delirium tremens

A is an acute organic psychosis
B is due to neuronal degeneration caused by ethyl alcohol
C is due to neuronal degeneration caused by vitamin B_1 lack
D is a complication of cirrhosis
E may be terminated by giving alcohol

Note: Delirium tremens may occur following withdrawal of alcohol from a dependent individual. It is characterised by anxiety, nausea, sweating, hallucinations, tremor and disturbed sleep. As the condition progresses seizures may occur, the subject becomes disoriented, weak, confused, and persecuted by his hallucinations.

A TRUE A psychosis is a condition in which the patient is out of touch with reality in a way that no healthy person can envisage. Confusion, clouding of consciousness and delirium are all characteristic. It is termed organic when the mental symptoms arise from verifiable physical causes, e.g. alcoholism. Acute organic conditions are by definition reversible, and no histopathological changes can be seen in the brain.

B FALSE Cerebellum and corpus callosum degeneration is known to occur in some chronic alcoholics, but the cause is unknown. It contributes to the alcoholic psychosis not that seen on withdrawal.

C FALSE Alcohol suppresses appetite and provides calories, and chronic alcoholics have a poor unbalanced diet that leads to multinutritional deficiencies. Thiamine (vitamin B_1) is one important substance that may be deficient and cerebral changes occur as a result, causing confusion, ocular palsy and ataxia (Wernicke's encephalopathy). Thiamine deficiency is not essential to the manifestation of delirium tremens.

D FALSE Consumption of large quantities of alcohol, particularly with an inadequate diet, produces hepatic damage. Cirrhosis is one of several changes that occur in the liver, which becomes tawny in colour due to diffuse hepatic fibrosis. It is associated with chronic alcohol consumption rather than withdrawal from it.

E TRUE The withdrawal syndrome to a drug of dependence can be terminated by giving the agent on which the individual is dependent. Thus delirium tremens may be controlled by giving alcohol.

211 Individuals who are morphine addicts typically show

    A a tolerance to the effects of morphine
    B pin-point pupils
    C a withdrawal response following administration of naloxone
    D convulsions on withdrawal
    E cirrhosis of the liver

A TRUE Tolerance is the term given to a diminishing response following repeated administrations of a drug, and one of the characteristics of addiction is the development of tolerance with the consequent desire to increase the dose in order to obtain a similar response. Tolerance does not develop equally or at the same rate to all the effects of morphine, and addicts continue to show miosis (see B) and constipation, even when the other actions of the drug are less apparent. The tolerance is partly due to a more rapid metabolism of morphine and partly to a changed receptor response.

B TRUE By stimulating the IIIrd nerve nucleus, morphine induces pupillary constriction and enhances the pupillary response to light so that miosis occurs even in darkness. There is little tolerance to this effect and pin-point pupils are characteristic of addicts. Only when asphyxia occurs (e.g. following inhalation of vomit) will mydriasis take place.

C TRUE Naloxone is a competitive antagonist which if injected into morphine addicts will compete with the morphine for the opiate receptor site: the individual is effectively deprived of morphine and a withdrawal syndrome is precipitated within a few minutes, reaching a peak within half an hour. The withdrawal is more intense than that which follows abstinence, and although this technique has been used to diagnose morphine addicts it is an unnecessarily unpleasant procedure which should be avoided.

D FALSE Convulsions are a serious complication of withdrawal of alcohol and of barbiturates from dependent subjects, but do not occur when morphine is withdrawn from addicts.

E FALSE Many drugs and industrial chemicals can cause liver damage but the incidence of cirrhosis from this cause is small. In Europe and the USA the vast majority of cirrhosis cases occur in chronic alcoholics. It does not occur in morphine addicts, although hepatitis is likely due to unhygienic injection procedures.

212 Characteristically, persons who are addicted to morphine or other opiates

    A were first prescribed the drug by a doctor
    B are taking other dependence producing drugs
    C have developed tolerance to the euphoric effects of the drug
    D are only psychologically dependent
    E are overweight

A FALSE Many patients have become dependent on barbiturates and amphetamine following their prescription by a doctor, for the treatment of a medical condition. However, opiate addicts have generally been introduced to drug taking by acquaintances or pushers; in either event from illegal sources.

B TRUE Opiate addicts cannot always obtain or afford the drug of their choice and they frequently consume other agents in an attempt to deaden the worst aspects of withdrawal. Sometimes they also take stimulants like cocaine to overcome the hypnotic action of the opiate, and sometimes they simply consume the second drug unwittingly because it has been added to the opiate to dilute it and make a greater profit for the dealer.

C TRUE Both patients and addicts who receive opiates over a period of time become tolerant to their effects. This becomes expensive for the addict who needs to buy more and more to satisfy his craving. The tolerance is thought to be due in part to an increased rate of degradation and in part to adaptation to its effects in the cns (perhaps altered enkephalin turnover).

D FALSE Psychological dependence indicates a desire to continue taking a drug, but with no tendency to increase the dose (tolerance) and no withdrawal syndrome when the drug is stopped. These are physical signs of dependence and are characteristic of opiate dependence.

E FALSE Opiate addicts are likely to spend a major part of their daily life in procuring, taking and recovering from their drugs. Most of their money is spent on drugs so that their accommodation is the cheapest obtainable, often squalid and insanitary. They neglect their personal hygiene and eat inadequately and irregularly. They often suffer therefore from ill-health and are commonly underweight.

213 Uterine relaxation may be induced by

    A salbutamol
    B ethyl alcohol
    C prostaglandin E_2
    D oxytocin
    E progesterone

A TRUE By stimulating β_2-receptors, intravenous infusion of salbutamol produces a uterine relaxation which may help to prevent premature labour.

B TRUE Ethyl alcohol produces relaxation of the uterus in two ways. Firstly, it has a direct action on the uterine smooth muscle, and secondly, it inhibits oxytocin secretion from the pituitary; both reduce the tone of the uterus. The use of alcohol during pregnancy is not recommended, however, because there is evidence that it may cause fetal damage.

C FALSE Prostaglandin E_2 is a myometrial stimulant and can be used to induce abortion or to promote labour.

D FALSE Oxytocin is the polypeptide hormone released from the neurohypophysis in response to suckling. This brings about milk ejection, although at the same time uterine contractions may occur. Oxytocin is also released during pregnancy and during the last few weeks before labour the myometrium becomes increasingly sensitive to the stimulant effects of oxytocin. The precise role of oxytocin in the physiology of labour is still not clear, but oxytocin, when given by intravenous infusion, is a useful method of inducing labour.

E TRUE Progesterone causes hyperpolarisation of the membrane of myometrial cells which has the effect of reducing their excitability (i.e. relaxation occurs). It has been suggested that a fall in progesterone levels at term may be contributory in effecting labour contractions.

214 The uterine myometrium at term is

A relaxed by halothane
B contracted by progesterone
C unaffected by orally administered ergometrine
D relaxed by nitrous oxide
E insensitive to prostaglandin $F_{2\alpha}$

A TRUE Halothane strongly inhibits myometrial tone and strongly inhibits the responses to both ergometrine and oxytocin. It should be employed with caution during delivery.

B FALSE Progesterone by hyperpolarising the myometrial cell membrane reduces its excitability and thus its response to uterine stimulants. In fact, the fall in circulating progesterone levels at term may contribute to the initiation of uterine labour contractions.

C FALSE Ergometrine produces a profound uterine contraction following oral administration, but it is not given to induce labour because of the increase in basal uterine tone that occurs. It is used to control postpartum haemorrhage.

D FALSE Nitrous oxide is commonly administered during labour as a 50 : 50 combination with oxygen. Excellent analgesia is achieved without decreasing either maternal oxygen saturation or uterine contractions.

E FALSE Prostaglandins E_2 and $F_{2\alpha}$ produce profound stimulation of the uterus throughout pregnancy and can be used to induce second trimester abortions or to induce labour.

215 In combined oral contraceptives, oestrogens

    A inhibit release of luteinising hormone (LH)
    B inhibit release of follicle stimulating hormone (FSH)
    C cause increased risk of blood clotting
    D cause thickening of cervical mucus
    E inhibit ovulation

A FALSE During the normal menstrual cycle, as the follicle develops, there is a rise in the level of circulating oestrogen which triggers a sudden discharge of LH from the pituitary. In the combined pill such a surge of gonadotrophin secretion does not occur. However, the suppression of LH is thought to be due to the progestogen (not the oestrogen) component of the pill.

B TRUE The action of oestrogen during the preovulatory phase of the menstrual cycle is to reduce FSH secretion by feed back inhibition on the hypothalamus. In the combined pill, the oestrogen component has a similar action, so that there is only a basal secretion of FSH throughout the period of administration.

C TRUE Patients receiving oestrogens or combined oral contraceptives have been shown to have accelerated blood clotting, increased levels of clotting factors in the blood, and increased platelet aggregation. The precise relationship of these findings to the increased risk of thromboembolic incidents in such patients is still obscure.

D FALSE An abundant watery secretion is produced by the cervix under the influence of oestrogens at ovulation, and is generally regarded as essential to the wellbeing of the sperm. Thick, tenacious cervical mucus is a characteristic of the combined contraceptive and is thought to impair sperm penetration. It is an anti-oestrogenic effect of the progestogen component.

E FALSE By reducing FSH secretion (see B) oestrogens inhibit follicular development and thus suppress ovulation. They are not used by themselves but in combination with progestogens, which assist in preventing ovulation.

216 In oral contraceptives, progestogens

A inhibit release of luteinising hormone (LH)
B inhibit release of follicle stimulating hormone (FSH)
C cause increased risk of blood clotting
D cause thickening of cervical mucus
E inhibit ovulation

A TRUE The progesterone release during the luteal phase of the normal cycle leads to a secretory endometrium, and the abrupt decline in progesterone release is the main factor in precipitating menstruation. Circulating progesterone inhibits LH secretion and this may be sufficient by itself to inhibit ovulation, e.g. during pregnancy. Inhibition of LH secretion and thus ovulation also occurs with synthetic progestogens such as medroxy progesterone.

B FALSE FSH release from the pituitary is effected by gonadotrophin releasing hormone (GnRH) from the hypothalamus. High circulating oestrogen levels, by an action on the hypothalamus, reduce GnRH secretion and thus FSH output. However, progestogens do not affect FSH secretion.

C FALSE Increased blood clotting is a characteristic of the oestrogen component of the combined pill, not the progestogenic component.

D TRUE Under the influence of progestogens, cervical mucus becomes viscous and tenacious, and provides an almost impenetrable barrier to sperm penetration.

E TRUE By suppressing the surge in LH secretion from the pituitary (see A), progestogens inhibit ovulation, and although they can be used alone as contraceptives addition of oestrogens makes them more reliable and helps to prevent breakthrough bleeding (see opposite, Q215E).

217 In the classical combined oral contraceptives

   A the oestrogen component inhibits breakthrough bleeding

   B the progestogen component inhibits ovulation

   C endogenous secretions of follicle stimulating hormone (FSH) and luteinising hormone (LH) are increased

   D the progestogen component is largely responsible for the thromboembolic side effects

   E the risks associated with their use are higher in women under 35 years of age than in those over 35 years

---

A TRUE   If progestogens are used alone as contraceptives (see B), proliferation of the endometrium occurs which then becomes unstable, so that breakthrough bleeding may occur. Addition of oestrogen prevents this from happening.

B TRUE   By suppressing circulating LH levels, and in particular the surge in level that precedes ovulation (see C), the progestogen component of the oral contraceptive will help to inhibit ovulation. Progestogens can be used by themselves as contraceptives (e.g. chlormadinone), but ovulation is not prevented in every cycle, and erratic endometrial bleeding may occur.

C FALSE   Measurements of circulating FSH and LH show that oestrogen-progestogen combinations suppress the levels of both hormones. They do this by an action on the hypothalamus to reduce the output of gonadotrophin releasing hormone and hence the secretion of FSH and LH from the pituitary. There may also be a direct action on the pituitary to reduce its sensitivity to the hypothalamic releasing hormone.

D FALSE   It is the oestrogen, not the progestogen component of the pill, that increases the risk of thromboembolic complications. The introduction of pills with minimal oestrogen content (< 50 μg/day) has considerably lowered but not totally abolished this risk.

E FALSE   The mortality and morbidity associated with use of the pill increases with increasing age, and it is now generally agreed that above the age of 35 these risks become more significant especially in smokers, and that alternative means of contraception should be used.

218 The classical combined oral contraceptives

    A inhibit follicular development
    B may increase hyperglycaemia
    C inhibit penetration of sperm into the uterus
    D make cervical mucus more viscous
    E produce a pseudodecidualised endometrium

A TRUE The oestrogen component of the combined pill has an action on the hypothalamus (via the gonadotrophin releasing hormone) to reduce the secretion of follicle stimulating hormone (FSH) from the pituitary. Only basal levels of FSH are detectable in the plasma with none of the peaks of the normal cycle. This prevents follicular development.

B TRUE The oestrogen component of the contraceptive pill has a complex action on carbohydrate metabolism that results in a decreased glucose tolerance which may aggravate diabetes. The contributing factors include antagonism of insulin action, increased blood levels of insulin and adrenal cortical hypertrophy.

C TRUE See D.

D TRUE Under the influence of the progesterone component of the combined pill, the cervical mucus becomes thick and tenacious (normally it is watery). This provides an almost impenetrable barrier to sperm penetration.

E TRUE In order that implantation can occur, the uterine endometrium must be in the correct stage of development. In the normal cycle, this is ensured by the sequential actions of oestrogen followed by progestogen. After use of the combined contraceptive pill, the secretory phase is reduced and a pseudodecidual reaction may occur, so that even if fertilisation takes place, it is unlikely that implantation would be successful.

219 Which of the following are recognised side effects of oral contraceptives

    A nausea
    B breast tenderness
    C weight loss
    D increased incidence of venous thrombosis
    E hypertension

A TRUE Nausea (and occasionally vomiting) resembling that which occurs early in pregnancy is a well recognised action of the pill. It is most apparent during the first month of use, but is rarely so bad as to prevent continued use. It is attributed to the oestrogen component, and is less troublesome in pills with low oestrogen content.

B TRUE Discomfort, tightness or tenderness of the breasts may accompany use of the pill. It is apparently due to the retention of salt and water caused by the oestrogen component.

C FALSE A gain in body weight of up to 1 kg is a common feature of the pill. It is attributed to the slight salt and water retaining properties of the oestrogen component.

D TRUE Studies in women taking the contraceptive pill have shown the incidence of deep vein thrombosis to be 5 to 6 times that in non-users. However, many of these women had taken pills containing more than 50 μg of oestrogen. If the amount of oestrogen does not exceed 50 μg/pill (the currently available pills are of this type), then the incidence is reduced by at least 25 per cent.

E TRUE The incidence of hypertension following prolonged use of oral contraceptives exceeds that in non-users. However, most studies show the excess incidence to be very small (certainly less than 2 per cent), but to increase with duration of use. The mechanism is not known, but may be due to changes in the renin-angiotensin-aldosterone system brought about by the progestogen component.

220 Which of the following drugs have been shown to interact with the combined oral contraceptives

    A warfarin
    B rifampicin
    C aspirin
    D diazepam
    E hyoscine

A TRUE Coumarin anticoagulants, like warfarin, act by inhibiting the synthesis of vitamin-K dependent clotting factors (II, VII, IX and X). Oral contraceptives increase the plasma levels of certain clotting factors, notably Factor VII and have been reported to reduce the effectiveness of oral anticoagulants.

B TRUE The incidence of breakthrough bleeding increases and a number of pregnancies have been reported in women who have taken rifampicin whilst using oral contraceptives. Rifampicin increases the hepatic metabolism of various drugs including the contraceptive steroids.

C FALSE No important interactions between aspirin and the oral contraceptives have been reported.

D FALSE Drugs that induce liver microsomal enzymes might be expected to reduce the efficacy of oral contraceptives. However, diazepam only does so very weakly and no important interactions with oral contraceptives have been reported.

E FALSE There have been no reports of interaction with hyoscine. However, this drug is widely used to treat motion sickness, and vomiting is recognised as a condition in which the contraceptive may become ineffective (because of inadequate absorption).

221 Which of the following drugs may be used to stimulate ovulation in infertile women

    A ethinyl oestradiol
    B clomiphene
    C bromocriptine
    D follicle stimulating hormone (FSH)
    E luteinising hormone (LH)

A FALSE Ethinyl oestradiol is a synthetic oestrogen with actions and uses similar to oestradiol. It is therefore used to treat primary amenorrhoea, to suppress lactation, to control menopausal symptoms and in combination with progestational agents, such as norethisterone, as an oral contraceptive.

B TRUE Clomiphene is an anti-oestrogen that stimulates the hypothalamic-pituitary axis to secrete gonadotrophic hormones. The increased gonadotrophin secretions may, if correctly timed, induce ovulation. This drug will only be effective if the hypothalamic-pituitary-ovarian axis is intact.

C TRUE Bromocriptine stimulates dopaminergic receptors, the effect of which is to cause inhibition of the release of prolactin by the pituitary with a consequent fall in circulating prolactin levels. Hypogonadism, amenorrhoea and infertility due to hyperprolactinaemia can thus be treated successfully with this drug.

D TRUE Human FSH can be obtained in a semi-purified and standardised form from either the urine of postmenopausal women, or from pituitary glands. It contains some LH. It is given by intramuscular injection to women in the treatment of anovulatory infertility (due to absent or low gonadotrophin secretion). Its effect is to induce follicular maturation and endometrial proliferation, but because this may not be complete it is common to give in addition chorionic gonadotrophin to stimulate ovulation and corpus luteum formation.

E TRUE LH is extracted from the pituitary or urine of postmenopausal women. It is used with human FSH (see D) to induce follicular maturation in women whose infertility is due to failure of ovulation because of inadequate gonadotrophin levels. Chorionic gonadotrophin (extracted from the urine of pregnant women) has similar actions.

Endocrines — Reproductive system: related question 109

222 Thyroid stimulating hormone (TSH)

A is released in response to cold
B is released in response to lowered blood thyroxine levels
C displaces circulating thyroxine from protein-binding sites
D causes release of calcitonin
E increases growth and vascularity of the thyroid gland

A TRUE Exposure to cold initiates a response through higher centres of the brain to bring about stimulation of the hypothalamus and release of the tripeptide, thyrotrophin releasing hormone (TRH), into the capillaries that supply the anterior lobe of the pituitary. This evokes release of TSH.

B TRUE The basal secretion of TSH from the anterior pituitary is controlled by the level of hormone to which this gland is exposed and a fall in the circulating level of unbound thyroxine initiates an increase in TSH output (i.e. a negative feed back system is operating).

C FALSE Thyroxine is strongly bound to circulating plasma protein especially thyroxine-binding globulin and less than 0.1 per cent is free in the circulation. The thyroxine may be displaced by various drugs, including aspirin, but this has little long term effect, in that the increase in free hormone mediates reduced TSH output from the pituitary (see B). TSH which is a glycoprotein with a molecular weight of 33,000 does not modify thyroxine binding.

D FALSE Calcitonin is a polypeptide which can be extracted from the thyroid gland. However, its secretion is not controlled by trophic hormones from the pituitary but by the calcium ion concentration of the extracellular fluid.

E TRUE A rise in the circulating level of TSH (following injection of this hormone or induced by cold stress) initially causes the acinar cells of the follicles to hypertrophy, and the colloid to be resorbed in order that the stored thyroxine can be liberated from the thyroglobulin and released into the circulation. If stimulation persists then the cells become columnar in shape and the whole gland becomes enlarged and highly vascular.

223 Thyroid hormones are

A polypeptides
B bound to albumin in the circulation
C bound to globulin in the circulation
D conjugated in the liver
E excreted in the bile

A FALSE In the synthesis of thyroid hormones, the starting material is a globulin. Tyrosine components of this are first iodinated to produce mono- and then di-iodotyrosine and, whilst still attached to the thyroglobulin, appropriate combination takes place to give tri-iodotyrosine (T_3) and thyroxine (T_4). Although produced from two amino acid molecules the thyroid hormones are not, however, polypeptides (i.e. are not linked by a peptide bond – CO.NH –), but have the following structure:

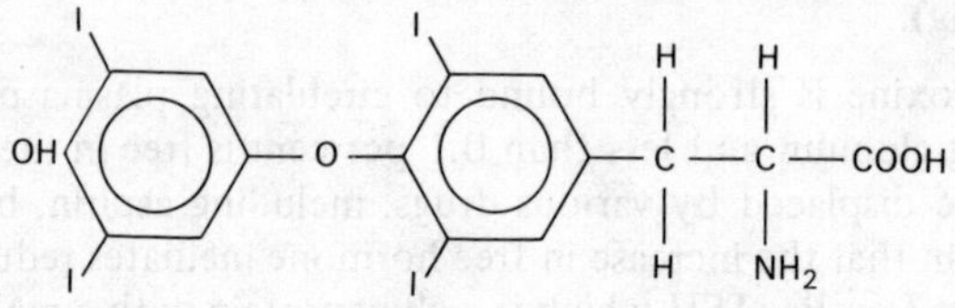

thyroxine

B TRUE A so-called thyroxine-binding prealbumin is present in the plasma. It binds both T_3 and T_4 but less avidly than the globulin carrier (see C). Its quantitative importance is difficult to assess.

C TRUE Thyroxine-binding globulin is the major carrier protein for circulating thyroid hormones. It is an acidic glycoprotein with a molecular weight of about 40,000, each molecule of protein binding one molecule of thyroxine (or T_3). As a result of binding less than 0.1 per cent of thyroxine and less than 0.4 per cent of T_3 in the plasma are free to produce a physiological action.

D TRUE The main route of metabolism of both T_3 and T_4 is through the liver where they are conjugated with glucuronic and sulphuric acids. The hormones are eliminated slowly, T_3 having a half-life of around 2 days and T_4 a half-life of about 6 to 7 days.

E TRUE The conjugates of thyroid hormone metabolism (see D) are excreted in the bile. Hydrolysis in the gut will then liberate some free compound which will be reabsorbed and return to the liver, i.e. enterohepatic circulation occurs. Nevertheless a significant proportion of the hormones is excreted in the faeces (in man between 20 to 40 per cent).

224 Thyroxine (T_4) is

    A stored intracellularly in the thyroid gland

    B present in the circulation in a greater concentration than tri-iodothyro-nine (T_3)

    C more powerful than T_3 (on a weight basis)

    D bound more strongly than T_3 to thyroxine-binding globulin

    E active in the bound form

A FALSE The thyroid gland is composed of follicles which are spherical in structure in which a layer of cuboidal epithelial cells surround and enclose a colloid. The thyroid hormones are synthesised in the cell by iodination of tyrosine components

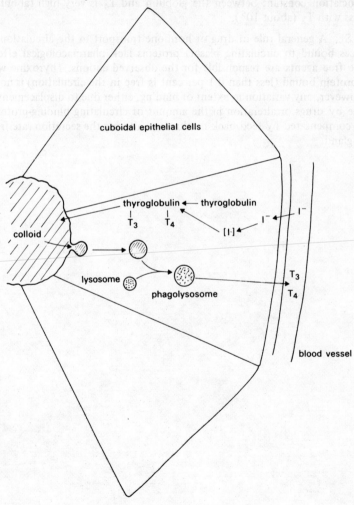

of a globulin. This thyroglobulin with the attached thyroxine (T_4) and T_3 is secreted from the cell into the colloid portion of the structure where it remains until required for secretion. Microvilli of the cell then engulf the thyroglobulin and following fusion with lysosomes the thyroid hormones are liberated and able to enter the circulation.

B TRUE In euthyroid individuals T_4 is present in the plasma at a level of 75 to 150 nmol/l whilst T_3 is present at a concentration of 1.1 to 2.2 nmol/l.

C FALSE It is generally estimated that T_3 is about four times as potent as T_4.

D TRUE Thyroid hormones in the circulation are carried principally by thyroxine-binding globulin, one molecule of protein binding one molecule of hormone. The association constant between the globulin and T_4 is very high (about 10^{10}), but is less with T_3 (about 10^6).

E FALSE A general rule of drug or hormone transport in the circulation is that substances bound to circulating plasma proteins lack pharmacological effect and only the free agents are responsible for the observed actions. Thyroxine which is highly protein bound (less than 0.1 per cent is free in the circulation) is no exception. However, any variation in extent of binding, either due to displacement of the hormone by drugs or alteration in the amount of circulating binding-proteins, are quickly compensated by feed back mechanisms altering the secretion rate from the thyroid gland.

225 The toxicity of thyroxine includes

A intolerance to heat
B diarrhoea
C precipitation of angina pectoris
D tremor
E anorexia

A TRUE Excessive amounts of thyroxine by stimulating basal metabolism are calorigenic and may cause slight pyrexia. As a consequence, the patients become warm and flushed and show an intolerance to heat.

B TRUE Increased gastrointestinal activity with resulting diarrhoea and perhaps malabsorption of nutrients may be a presenting feature in hyperthyroid patients. It also occurs when excessive amounts of thyroxine are administered to treat thyroid insufficiency.

C TRUE Peripheral vasodilatation, tachycardia and disorders of cardiac rhythm, such as extrasystoles and atrial fibrillation, are common cardiovascular manifestations of thyroxine excess. The effects on the heart are mediated at least in part by increased responsiveness to circulating catecholamines and to sympathetic nerve stimulation. In patients with latent ischaemic heart disease the excess thyroxine may increase heart work sufficiently to induce angina pectoris.

D TRUE A fine tremor of the fingers when the hands are outstretched is often seen in patients showing thyroxine toxicity, and is related to increased neuromuscular excitability and a change in the time course of the stretch reflex.

E FALSE As the metabolic rate rises and energy expenditure increases, so the appetite is stimulated. However, the additional intake of food is usually insufficient to compensate and patients lose weight.

226 Which of the following will diminish the signs of hypothyroidism

    A thyroxine (T_4)
    B tri-iodothyronine (T_3)
    C thyrocalcitonin
    D thiouracil
    E radioactive iodide (^{131}I)

A TRUE Two preparations of thyroxine are available for clinical use; d-thyroxine which is mainly used to lower blood cholesterol level and has little effect on basal metabolic rate, and l-thyroxine (T_4) which is the isomer secreted from the thyroid gland. The latter is given orally in the treatment of thyroid deficiency states but it has a delayed effect and cumulative action, and care must be taken initially to achieve the correct balance.

B TRUE Liothryonine sodium is the preparation of T_3 available for clinical use. It binds to plasma protein less readily than T_4, is more potent, acts more quickly (within a few hours) and has a shorter half-life. It is used when rapid treatment of a hypothyroid condition is required.

C FALSE Thyrocalcitonin is the alternative name for calcitonin, the polypeptide hormone that is secreted from the thyroid gland. It is involved in the control of calcium metabolism and its release is effected, not by trophic hormones from the pituitary but by the calcium ion concentration of the extracellular fluid.

D FALSE By inhibiting the iodination of tyrosine, thiouracil inhibits the synthesis of thyroid hormones and thus provides useful therapy for *hyper*thyroidism.

E FALSE Radioactive iodide (^{131}I) when used at a low level of activity (< 2 MBq) provides an excellent method for assessing thyroid function. In larger amounts (0.3 to 3 GBq) it may be used to destroy thyroid tissue and so is appropriate therapy in some cases of *hyper*thyroidism and malignant conditions of the thyroid gland.

227 Which of the following drugs may be useful in the treatment of hyperthyroidism

    A carbamazepine
    B radioactive iodide (^{131}I)
    C non-radioactive iodide
    D thyroxine (T_4)
    E propranolol

A FALSE Carbamazepine is a tricyclic compound related in structure to imipramine and the benzodiazepines. It is useful in the treatment of grand mal epilepsy, and trigeminal neuralgia.

B TRUE Radioactive iodine (^{131}I or ^{125}I), given as sodium iodide, is rapidly concentrated in the thyroid gland along with non-radioactive iodide. Small amounts (< 2 MBq) may be used for the assessment of thyroid function, but in order to destroy a portion of the gland in hyperthyroid patients between 100 and 500 MBq of ^{131}I are required.

C TRUE Lugol's solution, consisting of 5 per cent iodine, and 10 per cent potassium iodide has long been used in the therapy of hyperthyroidism, although of recent times its use has been largely confined to the treatment of thyroid crises and as a preoperative measure to reduce gland vascularity. The use of iodide in this situation is something of a paradox and the exact explanation of its efficacy is still being sought. It would appear that high intracellular levels of iodide inhibit the formation of both iodotyrosine and iodothyronine, perhaps by an action on the peroxidase enzyme which catalyses these reactions.

D FALSE Thyroxine (T_4) and tri-iodothyronine (T_3) are both liberated in excessive amounts in hyperthyroid patients and administration of further thyroxine would clearly exacerbate the condition.

E TRUE In hyperthyroid patients the heart rate is elevated (often over 100 beats/min), and abnormalities of cardiac rhythm may be apparent, e.g. extrasystoles and atrial fibrillation. This is due in part to direct stimulation of the heart muscle by the thyroid hormones, but also to increased sensitivity of adrenergic receptors to catecholamines released from sympathetic nerves or from the adrenal medulla. Propranolol by blocking β-adrenoceptors on the myocardium will help to reduce the palpitations and to protect against abnormal rhythms.

228 Thiouracils decrease thyroid function by inhibiting
    A iodine absorption from the gut
    B iodine trapping in the thyroid gland
    C iodination of tyrosine
    D the linking of di-iodotyrosine molecules
    E release of thyroxine from the gland

A FALSE Iodine enters the body as ionic iodide, elemental iodine or as iodine in organic combinations. It comes largely from the soil in which drinking water or foodstuffs originate, although a meal of sea fish will provide about a week's requirements. If it is present in the diet, it readily enters the body and ultimately the thyroid gland: there is no evidence of important drug interference with absorption.

B FALSE Iodine is largely reduced to iodide before absorption into the circulation. It then accumulates almost exclusively in the thyroid gland by a trapping mechanism which concentrates the iodide against a 25 : 1 gradient. Certain anions like thiocyanate and perchlorate are capable of inhibiting the energy-dependent process that brings about uptake but thiouracils have no effect at this site.

C TRUE Iodide trapped by cells of the thyroid must be converted to iodine before it can iodinate tyrosine. This oxidation is brought about by hydrogen peroxide made available from flavoproteins and catalysed by a peroxidase enzyme. The iodine produced by this process then interacts with tyrosine to give mono- and subsequently di-iodotyrosine. Thiouracils prevent the iodination of tyrosine probably by inhibiting the peroxidase enzyme, but other mechanisms such as interference with the flavoproteins to reduce the availability of hydrogen peroxide, or.binding to substrates, have not been ruled out.

D TRUE Coupling of mono- and di-iodotyrosine to form thyroxine (T_4) and tri-iodothyronine (T_3) is more sensitive to inhibition by thiouracil than the initial iodination process (see C). Peroxidase catalyses the coupling process as well as the iodination process and it is probable that thiouracil acts here also by inhibition of this enzyme.

E FALSE Thyroxine release from the gland is evoked by thyroid stimulating hormone (TSH) which also controls the overall activity of the thyroid cells. Antithyroid drugs do not interfere with this process.

229 Carbimazole diminishes thyroid function by

A preventing tri-iodothyronine (T_3) and thyroxine (T_4) release
B inhibiting formation of iodinated tyrosyl residues
C preventing iodine uptake by the gland
D producing thyroid atrophy
E inhibiting organic combination of iodine

A FALSE Although the levels of T_3 and T_4 in the thyroid gland will be diminished by treatment with carbimazole (see B), release of the existing hormone will be unaffected.

B TRUE Iodide trapped by the thyroid gland is converted to iodine before it can iodinate tyrosine. This oxidation process is effected by hydrogen peroxide made available by flavoproteins and catalysed by a peroxidase enzyme. The iodine then interacts with tyrosine residues of a globulin component within the cell to produce mono- and subsequently di-iodotyrosine. Carbimazole, in common with other thioamides (e.g. thiouracil), prevents the iodination of tyrosine, primarily by inhibiting the peroxidase enzyme, although other mechanisms such as interference with the production of hydrogen peroxide (H_2O_2) by flavoproteins and binding to substrates may also be involved.

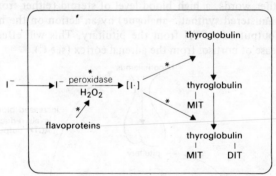

*Suggested sites of action of carbimazole

C FALSE Iodide accumulates in the thyroid gland against a considerable concentration gradient. An energy-dependent process is involved which is inhibited by perchlorate and thiocyanate but not by carbimazole.

D FALSE Quite the opposite, carbimazole may be described as goitrogenic. As the output of T_4 and T_3 from the gland falls (due to impaired synthesis) the low circulating levels will trigger release of thyroid stimulating hormone (TSH) from the pituitary. This in turn will act on the thyroid cells to induce the hyperplasia and increased vascularity characteristic of thyrotrophic stimulation.

E TRUE By inhibiting the availability of iodine (see B), carbimazole effectively inhibits organic binding of iodine to the thyroglobulin molecule and thus the formation of mono- and di-iodotyrosine.

230 Cortisol from the adrenal cortex

A is converted by the liver to hydrocortisone
B has mainly glucocorticoid (as opposed to mineralocorticoid) actions
C is secreted in response to a fall in circulating adrenocorticotrophic hormone (ACTH)
D increases in output when synthetic steroids are administered
E is synthesised from progesterone

A FALSE Hydrocortisone is simply an alternative name for cortisol. It is metabolised by the liver in part to produce cortisone.

B TRUE Cortisol affects both carbohydrate metabolism (glucocorticoid action) and salt and water metabolism (mineralocorticoid action). However, cortisol is much less potent than aldosterone as a mineralocorticoid and has about three times its glucocorticoid activity.

C FALSE The output of cortisol from the adrenal cortex increases in response to raised circulating levels of ACTH. The ACTH stimulates both synthesis and release of the steroid hormone.

D FALSE The output of ACTH from the pituitary is controlled by a negative feed back. In other words, a high blood level of steroid (either from the adrenal cortex or an administered synthetic analogue) by an action on the hypothalamus, will reduce the output of ACTH from the pituitary. This will effectively reduce synthesis and release of cortisol from the adrenal cortex (see C).

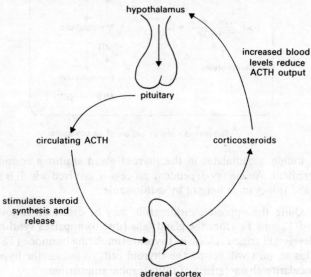

E TRUE The initial starting material for the synthesis of steroids in the body is cholesterol, but progesterone provides a common intermediate in the production of most steroid hormones including cortisol.

231 Glucocorticoids are clinically useful in the treatment of

A peptic ulcer
B ulcerative colitis
C acute leukaemia in children
D psychoses
E Cushing's disease

A FALSE Peptic ulceration is an occasional complication of glucocorticoid therapy which may be caused by delayed healing of pre-existing or aspirin-induced ulcers. In patients who already have peptic ulcers or who develop them during treatment, the use of steroids unless vital should be avoided.

B TRUE Patients with ulcerative colitis who do not respond to rest and a change of diet may require treatment with a glucocorticoid (e.g. prednisolone) given initially as a retention enema or, failing that, orally. The anti-inflammatory actions of the steroids appear to be responsible for their beneficial effects.

C TRUE Glucocorticoids reduce the ability of lymphocytes to undergo mitosis and are thus of value in the treatment of acute lymphoblastic leukaemia which is primarily a disease of children. Initial effects with prednisone and vincristine are striking with about 95 per cent of cases showing complete haematological remission.

D FALSE Nervousness, insomnia and mood changes are not uncommon during chronic treatment with glucocorticoids, and psychoses of the manic depressive or schizophrenic type may even occur. The most serious conditions develop in individuals with a previous history of psychosis.

E FALSE Cushing's disease is the name given to the syndrome characterised by moon-face, buffalo hump, skin thinning, muscle wasting, etc. caused by excessive blood levels of glucocorticoids. It may be due to a primary disorder of the adrenal gland, oversecretion of adrenocorticotrophic hormone (ACTH) from the pituitary, secretion of an ACTH-like peptide from another source, or simply due to the chronic systemic administration of large amounts of glucocorticoids for the treatment of another disease, e.g. rheumatoid arthritis.

232 Synthetic steroids like prednisolone

A are useful analgesics in the treatment of rheumatoid arthritis
B are anti-inflammatory
C cause diuresis
D cause dissolution of lymphoid tissue
E are useful in the treatment of severe chronic asthma

A FALSE Analgesics by definition are substances whose primary action is to prevent the initiation, transmission or perception of pain. The primary effect of prednisolone is anti-inflammatory, and only indirectly by reduction of local mediator release and joint swelling does it alleviate pain.

B TRUE Prednisolone and related steroids are amongst the most potent anti-inflammatory agents available. They have a complex mechanism of action which may include stabilisation of lysosomes, reduction of blood vessel permeability, and inhibition of mediator formation and recent evidence suggests that anti-inflammatory steroids may induce de novo synthesis of a polypeptide or protein which has antiphospholipase activity. This reduces the availability of arachidonic acid and hence the synthesis of prostaglandins (see diagram Q108, page 129).

C FALSE Prednisolone is not diuretic. If anything it has very slight mineralocorticoid action which would result in sodium and water retention, and oedema formation.

D TRUE All glucocorticoids will temporarily reduce the size of the thymus and other lymphoid tissues. For this reason they are of value in treating malignant conditions in these organs.

E TRUE Corticosteroids should not be used in the treatment of asthma until other measures have been shown to be ineffective. In severe chronic disease, however, their use may be life-saving. The mechanism of action is unclear, for there is no convincing evidence that in man they impair IgG or IgE formation, IgE binding to mast cells or the release of mediators from mast cells. Furthermore, the extent of their anti-inflammatory action does not always equate with the beneficial effects they induce.

233 Long term administration of prednisolone in humans characteristically causes

    A increased secretion of adrenocorticotrophic hormone (ACTH)
    B a reduced rate of wound healing
    C lowered resistance to infection
    D hypertension
    E suppression of antibody synthesis

A FALSE Secretion of ACTH from the pituitary increases as the level of circulating glucocorticoids falls, i.e. negative feed back occurs. An artificially high level of glucocorticoid following prednisolone administration conversely results in reduced ACTH secretion.

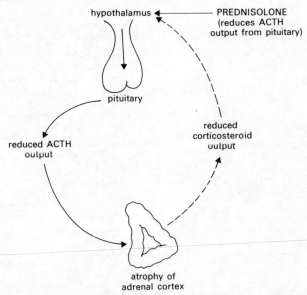

B TRUE The collagen content of the skin of patients treated with corticosteroids is much lower than in untreated patients, and skin damage occurs more frequently. This, coupled with a reduced inflammatory response and inhibition of fibrous tissue formation, causes an impairment of the rate of wound healing.

C TRUE By virtue of the reduced inflammatory response, both local and systemic responses to infection are reduced. This not only increases susceptibility to bacterial infections, but organisms which are not normally pathogenic in man may also invade the body, e.g. candida.

D TRUE Long term administration of a steroid that causes potassium depletion with sodium and water retention is likely to cause arterial hypertension; and although mineralocorticoid activity of prednisolone is not marked, hypertension does occur especially in patients with renal disease, and existing hypertension may be made worse. Patients receiving prolonged treatment with steroids should have their blood pressure checked at intervals.

E FALSE Although steroids like prenisolone are extremely useful in the control of allergic conditions like asthma there is no evidence in man that they significantly inhibit antibody formation. They may do so in some animals.

Endocrines — Adrenal cortex: related question 147

234 Insulin

A is a polypeptide
B for human use is extracted from pig pancreas
C is administered orally
D acts by enhancing cellular uptake of glucose
E acts by enhancing cellular utilisation of glucose

A TRUE Insulin is a polypeptide of molecular weight about 5,700 consisting of two parallel chains of amino acids joined by two S-S links.

B TRUE Both ox and pig pancreas provide the source of insulins for use in humans. Structurally, the pig insulin more closely resembles that from man, and it tends to be less antigenic.

C FALSE As with all polypeptides, insulin is destroyed by proteolytic digestive enzymes in the gastrointestinal tract. It is therefore given by injection, usually subcutaneously.

D TRUE The primary action of insulin in peripheral tissues is to increase the permeability of cell membranes to glucose, which then passes into the cell from the extracellular fluid mainly by active transport, but also by diffusion. The insulin binds to specific receptors on the membrane, but the precise mechanism by which it increases glucose transport remains unclear.

E TRUE Whilst it is true that the impaired glucose transport which occurs as a result of insulin lack in diabetics (see D) would be sufficient to explain the reduced glycogen production in these patients, there is evidence that insulin also controls directly the synthesis of glycogen. Its action is probably on the protein kinase system, adjusting the balance of metabolism so that glycogenolysis is inhibited and glucose conversion to glycogen is enhanced.

235 Blood glucose levels in a diabetic patient may be lowered by

    A smoking a cigarette
    B subcutaneous injection of adrenaline
    C administration of insulin
    D administration of glucagon
    E administration of codeine

A FALSE The nicotine absorbed from cigarette smoke produces stimulation of sympathetic and parasympathetic ganglia and release of adrenaline from the adrenal medulla. The adrenaline elevates blood glucose levels primarily by an action to increase cyclic AMP (cAMP) levels in liver cells (see B and diagram).

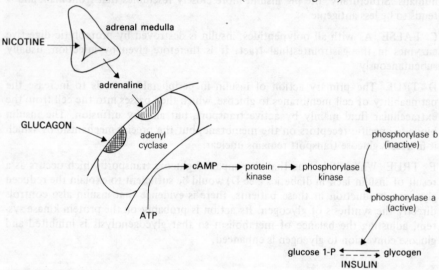

B FALSE Adrenaline has a complex metabolic action mediated primarily by stimulation of adenyl cyclase. This evokes a rise in cyclic AMP levels, which by activating phosphorylase in the liver and muscle brings about increased glycogenolysis. This and a concurrent reduction in glucose utilisation causes blood glucose levels to rise.

C TRUE Insulin decreases blood glucose in diabetic patients in at least two ways. It increases the permeability of cell membranes to glucose which thus passes from the extracellular fluid into the cell, but in addition it increases the conversion of glucose to glycogen.

D FALSE Administration of glucagon causes a rapid and immediate rise in the blood glucose level due mainly to activation of liver phosphorylase and the resulting glycogenolysis (see diagram).

E FALSE Whilst there is evidence that mild analgesics like aspirin and paracetamol may interfere with glucose metabolism, blood glucose levels are not significantly altered by clinical doses of codeine.

236 Blood clotting

    A in vitro is prevented by coumarin anticoagulants
    B is severely impaired in vitamin E deficiency
    C is prevented both in vivo and in vitro by heparin
    D is prevented by heparin principally by inhibition of the action of thrombin
    E is impaired by aspirin

A FALSE Anticoagulants of the coumarin type inhibit production in the liver of various clotting factors (II, VII, IX and X). There is a latent period of some 12 to 24 hours before they become effective, which relates in part to the half-life of these factors. Coumarins are ineffective in vitro.

B FALSE There is no good evidence that deficiency of vitamin E (which is a mixture of tocopherols) ever occurs in man, except in premature infants when increased haemolysis may result. Deficiency of vitamin K on the other hand rapidly leads to defective synthesis of clotting factors (especially prothrombin) by the liver and haemorrhages develop. This is rarely due to dietary deficiency, but rather to malabsorption or liver disease.

C TRUE Because heparin produces its anticoagulant effect mainly by inhibiting the action of thrombin (see D) it is effective both in vivo and in vitro.

D TRUE The principal action of heparin as an anticoagulant is to inhibit the action of thrombin, thus preventing the formation of fibrin.

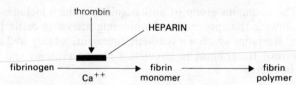

An α-globulin co-factor found in plasma is required for the heparin to be effective. Heparin also inhibits the formation of plasma thromboplastin.

E TRUE Aspirin has two actions which would inhibit blood clotting. First, it impairs the initial platelet aggregation that occurs in thrombus formation (by inhibiting the cyclo-oxygenase enzyme so that production of the potent platelet aggregator, thromboxane A_2 is reduced) and secondly, in high doses it inhibits prothrombin formation (possibly by competing with vitamin K in the liver — see B).

237 The anticoagulant warfarin

  A is added to blood which is to be used for transfusion to prevent coagulation
  B acts by reducing the production of thromboplastins
  C is found naturally in mast cells
  D has its action antagonised by protamine
  E is destroyed in the gastrointestinal tract

A FALSE Warfarin is only effective in vivo. It prevents blood clotting by interfering with the synthesis in the liver of Factors II (prothombin), VII, IX and X. It appears to do this by competing with vitamin K which is a co-factor for the synthetic enzymes. It is ineffective when added to blood in vitro.

B TRUE The various factors necessary for the activation of the clotting mechanism are known as thromboplastins, and their production by the liver is inhibited by warfarin (see A).

C FALSE The anticoagulant heparin is found in the large dense granules of mast cells in combination with histamine. Warfarin is a synthetic chemical of the coumarin type, some of which are found naturally in plants.

D FALSE Protamines are strongly cationic proteins obtained from the sperm of certain fish. They combine readily with heparin (which is an anion) to neutralise its anticoagulant effect, but are not of value in overcoming the anticoagulant effect of warfarin. In fact at high doses protamine inhibits thromboplastin formation (see B).

E FALSE The coumarin group of anticoagulants (which includes warfarin) was discovered following the appearance of a bleeding disease in cattle fed with a fermented clover. Warfarin, which is a synthetic coumarin, is fairly well absorbed from the gastrointestinal tract, binds to circulating plasma proteins and becomes concentrated in the liver.

238 When a patient has been established on an effective dose of the coumarin anticoagulant, warfarin

    A administration of aspirin will reduce its efficacy
    B prolonged administration of barbiturates may cause haemorrhage
    C the majority of the circulating warfarin is bound to plasma albumin
    D foods containing tyramine should be avoided
    E digitalis toxicity will be enhanced

A FALSE Aspirin and other salicylates have a very high affinity for binding sites on circulating albumin, and drugs like warfarin will be displaced. This increases the plasma free concentration and thus amplifies the pharmacological action of warfarin.

B FALSE Barbiturates will, over a period of time, cause induction of liver microsomal enzymes. This not only increases the rate of metabolism of the barbiturate (and so causes tolerance) but also increases the rate of metabolism of other substances dependent on the same enzyme system for their detoxification. Warfarin is metabolised in this way and will thus have a reduced effect.

C TRUE About 98 per cent of circulating warfarin is bound to plasma albumin (see A).

D FALSE Foods containing tyramine should be avoided only during treatment with monoamine oxidase inhibitors. Tyramine inactivation is unaffected by warfarin treatment.

E FALSE Adverse effects have not been reported following the use of digitalis in patients already receiving warfarin.

Blood: related question 28

239 Sulphonamide antibacterial drugs

    A destroy the bacterial cell wall
    B are bacteriostatic
    C combine with pteridine
    D block utilisation of para-amino-benzoic acid (PABA)
    E prevent synthesis of folic acid

A FALSE Antibiotics that interfere with the cell wall (e.g. cycloserine, penicillins) do so by inhibiting synthesis of essential components of this structure. Only the natural agent lysosyme actively destroys the cell wall. Such cells swell and burst due to the osmotic gradient, i.e. the compounds are bactericidal. This is not an action of the sulphonamides (see B).

B TRUE Sulphonamides interfere with the production of folic acid (see E) which is essential for cell division. They therefore prevent bacterial multiplication, and allow the infection to be controlled by the normal homeostatic mechanisms of the body. They do not directly cause cell death and their action is described as bacteriostatic.

C TRUE Pteridine, together with PABA and glutamic acid, are essential precursors in the synthesis of folic acid by bacteria. Sulphonamides bind not only to pteridine but also to pteridine pyrophosphate (see diagram) to form an inactive complex, thus preventing its conversion to folic acid.

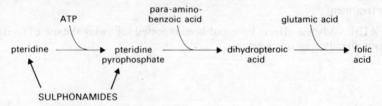

D TRUE The sulphonamides compete with PABA for binding sites on the pteridine. This is competitive antagonism and excess PABA will overcome the blockade.

E TRUE Most bacterial cells cannot utilise preformed folic acid and synthesise it as required from the basic components (see diagram). Sulphonamides inhibit such synthesis and thus reduce the availability of folinic acid which is an essential carrier of 1-carbon units in the synthesis of various substances, e.g. thymidylic acid, purines etc. Cells showing resistance to sulphonamides either do not require folate or can incorporate it directly.

240 Trimethoprim acts

A by blocking utilisation of para-amino-benzoic acid (PABA)
B by inhibiting bacterial dihydrofolate reductase more than animal dihydrofolate reductase
C by combining with 80s ribosomes
D as an antimetabolite
E to reduce the supply of 1-carbon units.

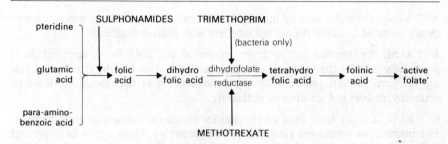

A FALSE The sulphonamides (not trimethoprim) competitively inhibit the utilisation of PABA in the synthesis of folic acid by bacterial cells.

B TRUE Folate reductase is present in both animal and bacterial cells, and although methotrexate will inhibit both, trimethoprim only inhibits the enzyme to any significant extent in bacterial cells: being about 60,000 times more effective against the bacterial enzyme. This is related to differences in the enzyme rather than problems of penetration or distribution.

C FALSE Trimethoprim does not bind to either mammalian (80s) or bacterial (70s) ribosomes, and does not interfere with protein synthesis.

D TRUE Any agent that inhibits the normal production of essential substances within the body may be described as an antimetabolite. They are usually agents that structurally resemble the appropriate precursor and are either incorporated to produce a false mediator or metabolite, or simply inhibit further synthesis by that pathway. Trimethoprim resembles the pteridine part of the folic acid molecule the metabolism of which it inhibits.

E TRUE 'Active folate' is the name given to the various forms in which tetra-hydrofolic acid is made available for the transfer of 1-carbon units in synthetic processes in bacteria and throughout the body. Trimethoprim by inhibiting folic acid metabolism will, therefore, interfere with the synthesis of purines, pyrimidines, thymidylic acid and a number of other biochemical pathways.

241 Which of the following drugs block protein synthesis by an action at the ribosomal level

    A penicillin
    B actinomycin D
    C tetracycline
    D chloramphenicol
    E cotrimoxazole

A FALSE Penicillin acts by interfering with cell wall synthesis to produce osmotically sensitive bacteria. It does not interfere with protein synthesis.

B FALSE By binding to the lesser groove of the DNA helix, actinomycin D powerfully inhibits the synthesis of messenger-RNA. This has the effect of inhibiting de novo protein synthesis by preventing coding at the ribosome. However, actinomycin does not act directly at this site.

C TRUE Tetracyclines bind to the smaller ribosomal subunit in both bacterial and mammalian ribosomes (30s and 40s respectively). Their action is to prevent the exchange of amino acids from transfer-RNA to the growing peptide chain, so that protein synthesis is effectively halted. They probably do this by preventing attachment of the transfer-RNA to the ribosome.

D TRUE This drug inhibits protein synthesis by binding to the 50s subunits of the 70s bacterial ribosomes. The overall effect is to cause release of part-formed peptides, and to inhibit further protein synthesis by preventing binding of messenger-RNA. Some 70s ribosomes are present in mammalian mitochondria which may explain some of the toxic effects of the drug.

E FALSE Cotrimoxazole is the name given to the combination of sulphamethoxazole and trimethoprim, drugs which interfere with the bacterial synthesis and utilisation of folic acid.

242 Streptomycin

  A inhibits protein synthesis
  B inhibits RNA polymerase
  C is an aminoglycoside antibiotic
  D has neuromuscular blocking activity
  E causes discolouration of the teeth if given during tooth calcification

---

A TRUE By binding to protein in the 30s subunit of bacterial ribosomes, strepto-mycin causes misreading of the messenger-RNA so that incorrect amino acids are incorporated into the growing peptide. This has the effect of inhibiting protein synthesis. The mistakes are not random and usually involve misreading of a purine.

B FALSE RNA polymerase is involved in the transcription of information from DNA to messenger-RNA, a process that is inhibited by agents that bind to the minor groove of the DNA helix, e.g. actinomycin D. It is not inhibited by strepto-mycin.

C TRUE Streptomycin was discovered following a systematic search for anti-biotics in soil fungi. A strain of *Streptomyces griseus* was shown to have anti-microbial activity and the drug now called streptomycin was isolated. Chemical analysis has since shown it to be an aminoglycoside.

D TRUE Respiratory difficulties may follow the postoperative instillation of streptomycin into the peritoneal cavity. This is due to the neuromuscular blocking action of the drug. Two mechanisms are thought to be involved, namely reduced acetylcholine release and reduced sensitivity of the postjunctional membrane. Patients receiving neuromuscular blocking drugs or who are myasthenic are parti-cularly sensitive.

E FALSE Toxic effects of streptomycin include hypersensitivity reactions, paraesthesias, vertigo, and cranial nerve deafness, but not discolouration of teeth. This is an effect seen with tetracyclines if given during tooth calcification.

243 Chloramphenicol affects bacterial cells selectively because it

    A only inhibits 70s and not 80s ribosomes

    B binds to bacterial single-stranded DNA

    C inhibits bacterial cell wall synthesis

    D cannot pass through mitochondrial membranes

    E cannot pass through plasma membranes

A TRUE 80s ribosomes are found in mammalian cells and unlike bacterial 70s ribosomes are unaffected by chloramphenicol. In bacteria, chloramphenicol binds to the 50s subunit to prevent proper attachment of the messenger-RNA and inhibit peptide bond formation so that part-formed peptides are released. The 70s ribosomes are not exclusive to bacteria, however, and are found in some mammalian mitochondria. Damage at this site is usually minimal (see D).

B FALSE Whilst inhibitors of nucleic acid synthesis like proflavine and actinomycin have been shown to bind to single-stranded DNA there is no evidence that this is an action of chloramphenicol.

C FALSE This is an action of the penicillins and cycloserine but not of chloramphenicol.

D TRUE The absence of any significant action of chloramphenicol on the 70s ribosomes in mammalian mitochondria is because the drug does not usually pass the mitochondrial membrane in large enough amounts to cause damage. However, toxicity of the drug, e.g. bone marrow depression, may be due to such an action.

E FALSE Although the plasma membrane does control to some extent the passage of substances into the cell, orally active drugs like chloramphenicol that can pass through membranes to enter the body will readily gain access to the cytoplasm of the cell. Only passage into the mitochondria may be restricted (see D).

244 The actions of penicillin include

A inhibition of bacterial cell wall synthesis
B destruction of mature bacterial cell wall
C arrest of protein synthesis
D inhibition of folic acid metabolism
E production of osmotically sensitive bacteria

A TRUE Bacterial cell walls have considerable strength and rigidity due to the nature and structure of the components. Essentially they consist of a mucopolysaccharide (frequently alternating units of N-acetyl glucosamine (NAG) and N-acetyl muramic acid (NAM)) with peptide side chains each of which is linked by peptide bonds or further short peptide chains. Penicillin inhibits the transpeptidase enzyme that is responsible for the formation of the peptide links between the mucopeptide molecules. (See also E)

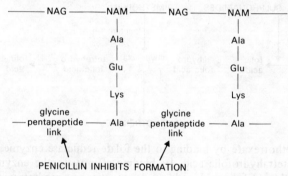

B FALSE Penicillin inhibits formation of the cell wall during normal growth, but will have no effect on the structurally intact mature cell. Growing cells that are insensitive to penicillins either have only limited mucopeptide in their cell walls or have walls that impede penicillin penetration.

C FALSE Antibiotics like tetracyclines, chloramphenicol, streptomycin and neomycin all significantly inhibit protein synthesis, but this is not an action of the penicillins.

D FALSE The antimetabolite, methotrexate, will interfere with folic acid metabolism, but this is not a site of action of penicillin.

E TRUE Bacterial cells have a high internal osmotic pressure (750 to 1000 mosmols). By reducing the structural integrity of the cell wall (see A) penicillin produces a cell that will swell and burst under the influence of the osmotic gradient. It will also become more sensitive to mechanical stress.

271

245 The conversion of folic acid to folinic acid

    A in human cells is inhibited by cytarabine
    B in bacterial cells is inhibited by sulphonamides
    C when inhibited by methotrexate can be restored by administering
       excess folic acid
    D is inhibited by alkylating agents
    E is inhibited in bacterial cells by trimethoprim

A FALSE Cytarabine is an antipyrimidine the most important effect of which is to inhibit DNA synthesis by an action on DNA polymerase.

B FALSE Sulphonamides, by competing with the structurally similar para-amino-benzoic acid, inhibit the synthesis of folic acid. They do not interfere with the conversion of folic acid to folinic acid.

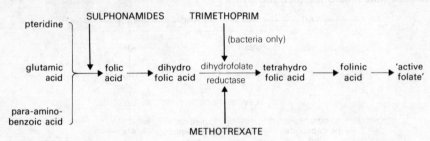

C FALSE Methotrexate by binding to the folate reductase enzyme, inhibits the production of tetrahydrofolic acid. Its binding affinity to the enzyme is almost 100,000 times that of folic acid, and in order to overcome methotrexate toxicity it is necessary to administer folinic acid (see diagram).

D FALSE Alkylating agents by binding to DNA interfere primarily with DNA replication.

E TRUE Dihydrofolate reductase is found in both bacterial and human cells, but trimethoprim will only inhibit the enzyme to any significant extent in bacterial cells. It is about 60,000 times more effective against bacterial folate reductase than against the human enzyme.

246 In the treatment of malignant diseases

    A fluorouracil is effective because it inhibits purine synthesis
    B daunorubicin is another name for actinomycin
    C cyclophosphamide is only effective after metabolic conversion
    D vinblastine arrests cell division in metaphase
    E asparaginase inhibits the production of asparagine

A FALSE Fluorouracil is an antipyrimidine that acts following metabolic conversion by inhibiting the synthesis of thymidylic acid, a supply of which is essential to normal DNA replication.

B FALSE These are two distinct antibiotics which have in common the ability to inhibit RNA polymerase. Actinomycin does this by hydrogen bonding to guanine units in the minor groove of DNA and daunorubicin by intercalation of the DNA.

C TRUE Cyclophosphamide is known as a 'latent mustard' and is not effective against tumour cells in vitro. To be effective in vivo it must first be metabolically activated by microsomal enzymes, primarily in the liver.

D TRUE Vinblastine by inhibiting spindle formation arrests cell division in metaphase. It probably does this by preventing the synthesis of microtubular proteins of the spindle.

E FALSE Some leukaemic cells are dependent on a plentiful supply of asparagine for their growth and replication. Asparaginase (colaspase) is effective in treating these tumours because it metabolises the asparagine. Resistance may subsequently develop as the malignant cells develop the ability to synthesise their asparagine requirement.

247 Which of the following cytotoxic drugs is/are antimetabolite(s)

A azathioprine
B mustine
C methotrexate
D mercaptopurine
E cortisol

Note: Antimetabolites are chemically similar to naturally occurring essential substances with which they compete for sites on various synthetic enzymes. They produce inhibition of enzyme activity and reduce incorporation of the natural precursors into the synthetic process. This impairs both cell growth and replication. The most important agents are purine, pyrimidine, glutamine and folic acid antagonists.

A TRUE Azathioprine is a purine analogue that is converted in vivo to mercapto-purine, which in turn interferes with purine metabolism (see D). It is used mainly as an immunosuppressant.

B FALSE As with all nitrogen mustards this substance is an effective inhibitor of cell division because it binds to the DNA strands to prevent their separation during replication. It is not classified as an antimetabolite but as an alkylating agent.

C TRUE Methotrexate is a folic acid antagonist which prevents the conversion of dihydrofolic acid to tetrahydrofolic acid by inhibiting the enzyme folate reductase. It has almost 100,000 times the affinity for this enzyme than the natural precursor, folic acid.

D TRUE It is an antipurine that acts by inhibiting a number of enzymes involved in normal purine metabolism.

E FALSE Cortisol is a naturally occurring corticosteroid which in pharmaco-logical amounts is useful in the treatment of malignant disease because it causes dissolution of lymph tissue. It is not an antimetabolite.

248 The alkylating agent cyclophosphamide used in the treatment of malignant disease

    A is more effective against tumours with short doubling times than those with long doubling times
    B causes immunosuppression
    C produces leucopaenia as a side effect
    D inhibits spindle formation
    E cross links guanine units of DNA

A TRUE Cyclophosphamide interferes with DNA replication (see E) and has an action primarily during the S-phase (i.e. DNA synthesis phase) of the cell cycle. It is only effective in cells undergoing division. The more frequent the division, i.e. the shorter the doubling time, the greater the effect it will have.

B TRUE Cytotoxic drugs prevent the increase in number of immunologically competent (antibody-producing) cells which normally follow an immune challenge, and have been used as immunosuppressants following organ transplantation.

C TRUE Cell division is inhibited by cytotoxic drugs at all sites throughout the body including the bone marrow. A fall in the number of circulating white cells (leucopaenia) may render the patient vulnerable to infection. Routine haematology is an essential part of treatment.

D FALSE Spindle poisons characteristically arrest cell division in metaphase by inhibiting spindle formation. They include colchicine, vinblastine and vincristine.

E TRUE Alkylating agents bind to the guanine units of DNA strands and when, as with cyclophosphamide, there are two alkylating groups, cross linkage between different DNA strands of the double helix will occur. Such an interaction interferes with separation of the strands during DNA replication.

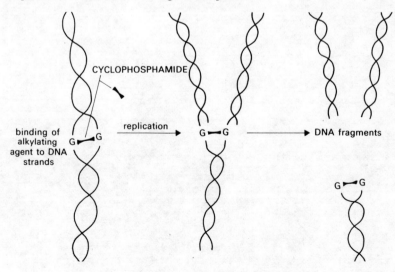

249 In the treatment of malignant disease, actinomycin D

    A competes with messenger-RNA for ribosomal binding sites
    B has a large therapeutic index
    C inhibits de novo protein synthesis
    D binds to DNA
    E inhibits the action of RNA polymerase

A FALSE A number of antibiotic drugs interfere with protein synthesis by bind-ing to the ribosome, and some like chloramphenicol compete with messenger-RNA for the binding sites. This is not the mechanism of action of actinomycin D (see D).

B FALSE The therapeutic index of a drug is the ratio of the maximum tolerated dose to the minimum effective dose; the larger the ratio, the safer the drug. Cyto-toxic drugs like actinomycin D are extremely toxic and have ratios approaching unity.

C TRUE See D.

D TRUE Actinomycin binds to DNA by hydrogen bonding in the minor groove. This has a number of effects, but predominant among them is that RNA poly-merase can no longer effectively read the information on the DNA; messenger-RNA production is blocked, and synthesis of new proteins is prevented.

E TRUE See D.

250 Which of the following are typically the result of treatment with cytotoxic drugs

A immunosuppression
B mental elation
C renal failure
D thrombocytopaenia
E leucopaenia

Note: Cytotoxic drugs as their name implies cause cell death. They are used mainly in the treatment of malignant disease and interfere primarily with the processes of cell replication. They prevent cell division throughout the whole body.

A TRUE By preventing the increase in numbers of immunocompetent (antibody-producing) cells that follows an immunological challenge, antibody synthesis is inhibited. Cytotoxic drugs like azathioprine have been used to suppress rejection following tissue transplantation and to treat rheumatoid arthritis.

B FALSE Cytotoxic drugs are all exceedingly toxic, but generally they have no direct effect on the cns. Depression as a consequence of the unpleasant side effect may be a more likely outcome than elation.

C FALSE Although some natural replacement of cells occurs in the kidney, it is not a site of rapid division, and cytotoxic drugs do not normally produce kidney damage, and certainly not sufficient to induce failure. Other toxicity would almost certainly prove fatal first.

D TRUE Interference with platelet production, and a fall in the peripheral count (thrombocytopaenia) is a common outcome of cytotoxic therapy, resulting in bleeding into the skin and elsewhere.

E TRUE A reduction in the number of all circulating blood cell types is expected following treatment and leucocytes are no exception. A fall in the number of white cells is particularly dangerous in that patients are very vulnerable to infection. Regular blood examination is an essential part of treatment.